The Prevention of Second Primary Cancers

Progress in Experimental Tumor Research

Vol. 40

Series Editor

Joseph R. Bertino New Brunswick, N.J.

The Prevention of Second Primary Cancers

A Resource for Clinicians and Health Managers

Hans Krueger Vancouver, B.C.
David McLean Vancouver, B.C.
Dan Williams Vancouver, B.C.

6 figures, 3 in color, and 75 tables, 2008

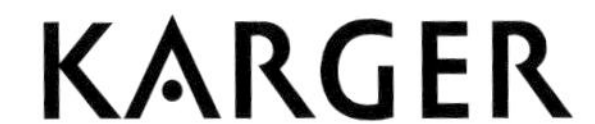

Basel · Freiburg · Paris · London · New York · Bangalore · Bangkok · Shanghai · Singapore · Tokyo · Sydney

Progress in Experimental Tumor Research
Founded 1960 by F. Homburger, Cambridge, Mass.

Hans Krueger, PhD
David McLean, MD
Dan Williams, MA
Cancer Prevention Programs
BC Cancer Agency
Vancouver, BC
Canada

Library of Congress Cataloging-in-Publication Data

Krueger, Hans.
The prevention of second primary cancers : a resource for clinicians and health managers / Hans Krueger, David McLean, Dan Williams.
p. ; cm. – (Progress in experimental tumor research, ISSN 0079–6263 ; v. 40)
Includes bibliographical references and index.
ISBN 978–3–8055–8497–5 (hard cover : alk. paper)
1. Cancer–Relapse–Prevention. I. McLean, David I., MD, FRCPC. II. Williams, Dan, 1957– III. Title. IV. Series
[DLNM: 1. Neoplasms, Second Primary–prevention & control. W1 PR668T v.40 2008 / QZ 200 936p 2008]
RC268.K74 2008
616.99'4–dc22

2008024733

Bibliographic Indices. This publication is listed in bibliographic services, including Current Contents®

www.karger.com
Printed in Switzerland on acid-free and non-aging paper (ISO 9706) by Reinhardt Druck, Basel
ISSN 0079–6263
ISBN 978–3–8055–8497–5
eISBN 978–3–8055–8498–2

This book is dedicated to Helena Krueger,
who died of a second primary cancer.

Contents

Krueger H, McLean D, Williams D: The Prevention of Second Primary Cancers.
Prog Exp Tumor Res. Basel, Karger, 2008, vol 40, pp 1–6

1

Overview of the Topic

So ist wohl auch die Annahme nicht auszuschliessen, dass, bei einem Individuum sich zweimal im Leben Carcinom entwickeln kann, wenn das erste mal radikale Heilung durch die Operation erzielt worden war. [We should probably not exclude the possibility that an individual can develop a second carcinoma even if an initial operation completely removed the first cancer.]

Theodore Bilroth, 1889.

This comment is found in a German report covering what were probably the first documented cases of second primary cancer (SPC) [1]. In the intervening 120 years, the research focus on this important area of oncology and epidemiology has been established and gradually intensified. Recently, investigation of prevention options has begun to dominate the agenda.

It is well known that cancer survivors are at risk for recurrence of the primary cancer. The chance of getting a so-called SPC is also increased. Simply put, a SPC is a new primary cancer developing in a person with a history of cancer. Interest in SPCs has paralleled the extraordinary improvement in curing primary cancers, which in turn has increased both the longevity and the absolute number of survivors. The concomitant reduction in mortality rates attached to (in particular) cardiovascular disease has augmented the general increase in longevity. Accordingly, the cumulative incidence of SPC has grown, essentially driven by patients surviving long enough for other cancers to develop. It is accurate to say that the SPC story has expanded as a by-product of increasing health awareness, early diagnosis of primary cancers and therapeutic success.

The outcome of these forces is that SPCs are now more common; indeed, as a class they are estimated to be the sixth most common form of malignancy in the world [2]. Consequently, research on such cancers has intensified. The last comprehensive textbook on the area covered data up to about 1997 [3]. It appears that the volume of publishing since that point has already matched the academic output in all the previous decades combined.

There are 3 imperatives that have prompted the continuing wave of research and analysis. First, there is a need to completely understand the epidemiology of SPC. This especially means evaluating the *excess* risk of developing a cancer when one has experienced a first primary. In other words, what is the increased chance of a cancer survivor getting any new cancer, or a particular type, compared to a random person from the general population? When expressed as a ratio of *observed* cancer incidence (among cancer survivors) over *expected* occurrences (in a general population), the resulting statistic is usually referred to as a Standardized Incidence Ratio (SIR). Although stated above in terms of individual risk, the statistic properly measures the excess risk across a group of people. For example, a SIR of 2.0 for leukemia means that double the number of leukemia cases will be observed among the cancer survivor cohort of interest compared with the same-sized control group drawn from the general population.

Next is the importance of knowing what might have precipitated any excess occurrence of cancer. In fact, studying SPC generation has proven to be a vital window onto the general topic of carcinogenesis in all types of tumors, whether or not they are first or second primaries.

Finally, there is the urgency to identify and test preventive measures that create a reduced risk of SPC, ideally at the level of individual survivors (the clinical agenda), and certainly across a group of survivors (the population health perspective). As we will see, preventive approaches might include decreased or mitigated use of potentially carcinogenic therapies, reductions in other risk factors, and appropriate screening and surveillance to detect and treat SPC as early as possible.

The Prevention of Second Primary Cancers is a synthesis of current research, culminating in pertinent summary charts (see chapter 15, pp 135–137), covering a whole spectrum of first and second primaries and the association between them. Naturally, all such results are selective, representing only the significant and substantial data. Since there are by some reckonings about 100 known cancers, a full accounting of every SIR would create a table approaching 10,000 cells.

What's in a Name?

The first task required in any overview of SPC involves understanding *exactly* how the term is applied in practice, in order that epidemiological results may be compiled and compared with confidence. The difficulty of this assignment is compounded by the wide variety of labels that more or less overlap with SPC. This makes conducting a comprehensive literature review particularly challenging.

The most common competing term is multiple primary cancer (MPC). The semantic distinctions between SPC and MPC are quite complex. For the purposes of this monograph, we will use MPC to cover all cases involving a plurality of cancers arising more or less independently from one another, *regardless of timing*. SPC, on the other hand, will be defined as neoplasms that arise independently in a new site or tissue and *subsequent* to the initial cancer, with the intervening period being at least 2 months in duration.

Epidemiology: State of the Art

Understanding the excess burden of *particular* SPCs is important in terms of focusing prevention efforts. Analysis of large cancer registries has consistently revealed that the SIR for all second cancers combined is less than 2.0; in some cases research has demonstrated no excess risk at all. Does that mean that there is no problem? Not at all. The story for specific SPCs also needs to be interpreted. The more detailed picture begins to reveal a compelling prevention agenda.

Measured across all patient ages, SIRs for particular first/second primary associations can be as high as 5.0. There are instances of dramatically higher risks reported in some studies, such as a SIR of about 16 for developing tongue cancer after laryngeal cancer [4]. In general, cancers located within the head and neck tend to show substantial linkages with first primaries. The report of associations within one region of the body (for example, a SIR of almost 34 for cancer of the small intestine following colorectal cancer, or 14 times the risk of vaginal cancer developing after cervical cancer) are perhaps not surprising. But what is one to make of a SIR of about 9 for leukemia following nasopharyngeal cancer?

Matters get even more pointed when age is taken into consideration. The literature shows that there are 2 themes in the SPC story that are serious for survivors of a childhood cancer such as Hodgkin's disease. First, the SIRs related to SPC can be very high, much higher than in the typical adult case of the same first primary. And second, the psychosocial impacts are particularly devastating: having survived the intense experience of a pediatric cancer, it is tragic to subsequently contract a second (and often fatal) malignancy.

In order to relevantly link both the psychosocial burden and the clinical urgency, we have organized the SPCs in each of our data tables in 2 ways, first, according to the potential years of life lost (PYLL) due to the second primary (an indication of population impact) and, secondly, by survival rate for each cancer (a measure of individual patient impact). Further, the 2 summaries of adult experience of SPC found at the end of the monograph (see chapter 15, pp 135–137) take into account both variables; they present the SPC information first in terms of descending prevalence and then by ascending survival. Again, by generally moving from more to less serious scenarios, we are attempting to present a picture of population and individual clinical priorities, and thereby to guide prevention efforts.

Etiology and Prevention

Three carcinogenic pathways have been confirmed with respect to SPCs. These comprise:

(1) a genetic factor common to the first and second primary
(2) an iatrogenic effect related to the treatment (whether radiation or chemotherapy) that is applied to the first cancer
(3) an environmental factor common to the first and second primary.

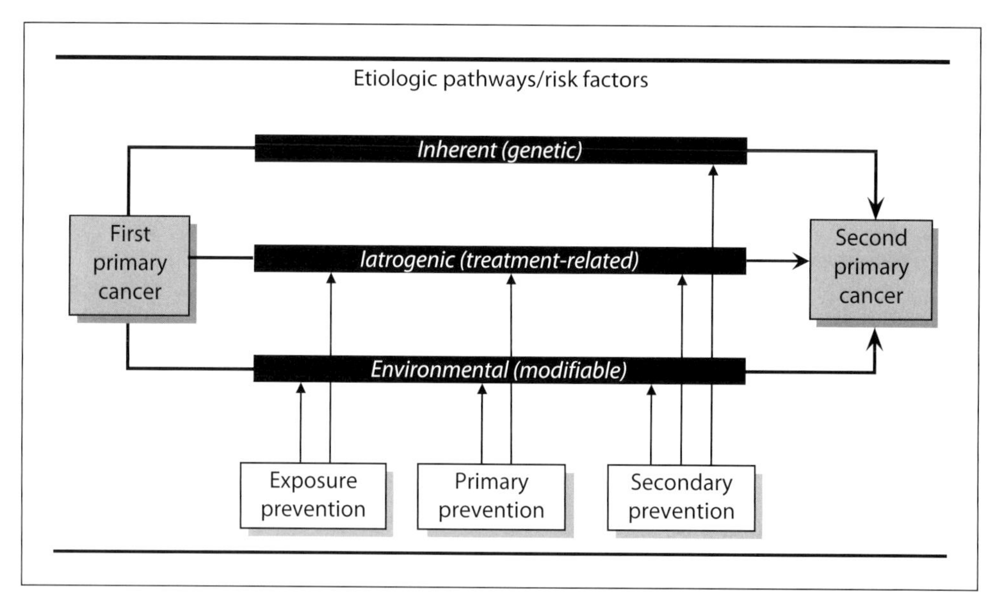

Fig. 1. Etiologic pathways/risk factors.

As indicated in the following chart, obvious primary prevention approaches arise with respect to the latter 2 pathways. Admittedly, the potential is limited in each case. First, it may be difficult to moderate treatment (and side effects) related to the first primary without lessening the cure rate. Second, whether the environmental factors are environmental in the colloquial sense (as in occupational or atmospheric exposures) or related to personal behaviors (as in smoking), the obstacles to change are often formidable. However, given time and innovation, all 3 carcinogenic pathways are potentially targetable (fig. 1).

Whatever the current limitations, it is important for both clinicians and population health leaders within the arena of cancer control to pay attention to prevention. This will include vigilance related to the onset or threat of any SPC. The aim, as always, is to detect any new cancer at an early stage when effective treatment is most possible. Sometimes, as in the case of pediatric cancer survivors, regular surveillance needs to be maintained for decades.

There is a growing sense that more should be done in this arena of cancer care and population health. While some topics may be reaching maturity, the intensity of research around new avenues for understanding and preventing SPC ought to be maintained. In particular, when SPC is an unfortunate by-product of the successful treatment of a first cancer, it is incumbent upon all concerned to look for safer cures in the future. As well, it is important to look for appropriate applications of new genetic insights and technologies that might be able to modify inherited risk factors.

In the meantime, while the breakthroughs are being sought, the serious business of careful follow-up and primary prevention must be focused on all cancer survivors at risk of SPC. A 3-point protocol for such patients would include:

(1) Opting for the least carcinogenic therapeutic agents or regimens available.

(2) Encouraging patients to modify potential risk factors that have a behavioral component. More than 50% of primary care deaths can be prevented by tobacco avoidance, a balanced diet, avoidance of obesity and exercise. Presumably, the same factors will apply to some types of SPC.

(3) Maintaining appropriate surveillance for SPC, to allow for early detection and treatment.

We will return to this protocol in the last chapter of this monograph. For now, we simply emphasize that the ultimate goal is to ensure that survivors of a first primary cancer, people that one researcher referred to (rather clinically) as 'natural experiments', experience as little physical suffering and mental distress as possible.

Purpose of this Project

To sum up, continued advances in cancer treatments have led to marked improvements in cure rates over the past 30 years. Longevity is also increasing through the control of risk factors such as tobacco use. At the same time, cancer survivors are at increased risk for recurrence of the primary cancer, as well as development of second primary malignancies. SPC has become an increasingly important concern in oncology during the last 2 decades. It is important from a clinical and prevention point of view to review and integrate the large volume of data that has emerged in recent years.

The goals of this book are:

(1) To review the current literature on SPC in order to gain an understanding of the epidemiology in general terms.

(2) To gain a good understanding of the excess risk of SPCs following an implicated first malignancy, both as a measure of the urgency of any prevention program and an indication of the potential benefits of such a program.

(3) To identify the known or suspected etiologic factors for SPCs, and to further narrow the field to those factors that are modifiable in practice.

(4) To note any effective preventive measures that might reduce the burden of SPC, both for individuals and across at-risk populations. The monograph seeks to provide guidance in terms of possibilities and priorities, to inform the work of clinicians and population health leaders.

We must begin by tackling in the next chapter this seemingly innocuous but actually quite complex question: what exactly is a SPC?

Notes and References

1 Quoted in Moertel CG: Multiple primary malignant neoplasms. Cancer 1977;40(suppl):1786–1792.

2 Callejo SA, Al-Khalifa S, Ozdal PC, et al: The risk of other primary cancer in patients with uveal melanoma: a retrospective cohort study of a Canadian population. Can J Ophthalmol 2004;39:397–402.

3 Neugut AI, Meadows AT, Robinson E (eds): Multiple Primary Cancers. Philadelphia, Lippincott Williams & Wilkins, 1999.

4 The examples in the introductory chapters are derived from specific studies that are detailed in the body of the monograph.

Krueger H, McLean D, Williams D: The Prevention of Second Primary Cancers.
Prog Exp Tumor Res. Basel, Karger, 2008, vol 40, pp 7–16

2

Meaning of SPC

Dimensions of a Definition

'The question is', said Alice, 'whether you can make words mean so many different things'. 'The question is', said Humpty Dumpty, 'which is to be master – that's all. They've a temper, some of them – particularly verbs, they're the proudest – adjectives you can do anything with, but not verbs – however, I can manage the whole lot of them!'

Lewis Carroll, Through the Looking-Glass, 1872

Medical terminology is often well characterized. However, because of many synonyms for the term and diverse 'near terms' used by those who publish on the topic, there are serious complexities associated with the definition of SPC.

The colloquial meaning is straightforward enough: an SPC is a new primary cancer in a person with a history of cancer. 'Primary' is a integral part of the definition; a primary cancer originates independently at a specific site in the body, rather than having spread to that location from another site [1]. It is distinguished from secondary cancer, where the primary disease has spread (metastasized) from the site in which it first appeared to a new site.

Although the terms are close (and, unfortunately, sometimes used in overlapping ways), it is most accurate and helpful to maintain a clear distinction between a SPC and a secondary cancer. The former is a new cancer, whereas the latter is an extension of an existing or previous cancer [2].

Defining the connection between cancers can ultimately involve analysis at the molecular level. For instance, metastases have a clonal relationship to the original cancer, that is, the cells involved in the 2 sites have an identical or near identical genetic make-up. Because of the obstacles that are sometimes present in identifying metastases, there is great interest in developing genetic tools to confirm the type of cancer that has been detected in each case. In other words, is it an old cancer revisited or a brand-new one? What is at stake is the fact that different preventive or therapeutic approaches are usually dependant upon whether the cancer of interest is a secondary or a second primary.

Problems emerge, however, in understanding precisely what 'new' means when applied to SPC. The question is an operational one for epidemiologists assembling databases or registries that track cancer incidence: how should emergent cancers be coded? When does a cancer qualify as a new entry in the registry? The definitional issue ultimately revolves around 2 dimensions, space and time.

First, there is the question of space, or the topography [3] of the cancer. A key question is whether a cancer is considered new when it occurs in the second of 2 paired organs (for example, kidneys, breasts) after appearing in the first organ of the pair. For the purpose of coding, the answer usually has been 'no'. A further question is as follows: does the term 'new' apply in any way to multifocal tumors, that is, 'discrete masses apparently not in continuity with other primary cancers originating in the *same* primary site or tissue'? [4] Again, for the purpose of epidemiological coding, the standard answer has been in the negative [5].

Next, we must consider if the cancer is truly new when it occurs in a *different* tissue type in the *same* organ. Here, the answer is 'maybe'. There are cancer experts that carefully consider such matters – often formed into working groups sponsored by organizations such as the International Association of Cancer Registries (IACR), based in Europe, and programs such as Surveillance Epidemiology and End Results (SEER) of the National Cancer Institute in the US. The rules developed by the IACR state that any cancer developing within certain histological types (including squamous carcinomas, basal cell carcinomas, adenocarcinomas and sarcomas) will be considered a new or different neoplasm [6]. On the other hand, a single cancerous type, such as lymphoma, leukemia, Kaposi sarcoma or mesothelioma, occurring in a systemic or multicentric form, is counted only once in any individual.

These sorts of guidelines represent only the broad brush strokes. The full picture concerning cancer registration is much more complex. For instance, the third edition of the SEER coding manual runs to 180 pages of detailed instructions, including all coding subsets. This raises an obvious question concerning how well any clinician or registry manager knows the manual and the detailed codes [7]. To aid this process, special attention has been paid in the literature to the specific criteria for SPC of the head and neck, the lung and the female breast. An illustration of the coding protocols is provided in the boxes on the following pages.

We must acknowledge that the dimension of timing is perhaps even more complicated. At this point, it is useful to reintroduce the main competing term in this area of oncology, that is, MPC. The application of this term in the literature is heterogeneous. MPC does not seem to be consistently used as a synonym for SPC, nor as a logical extension (that is, comprising second, third, etc. cancers as an overall class). For the most part, authorities are in agreement that MPC 'does not depend on time' [8]. In other words, it is a term used to describe an association without a sense of temporal direction, that is, to acknowledge 2 or more cancers in the same patient without reference to which one came first. This atemporality explains why 2 additional qualifiers are routinely used within the topic of MPC: synchronous and metachronous.

Box A: IARC Rules for Coding Multiple Primary Neoplasms [19]

(1) Recognition of the existence of 2 or more primary cancers does not depend on time.
(2) A primary cancer is one that originates in a primary site or tissue and is not an extension, recurrence or metastasis.
(3) Only 1 tumor shall be recognized as arising in an organ or pair of organs or a tissue. For tumors where the site is coded by the first edition of ICD-O (or by ICD-9), an organ or tissue is defined by the 3-character category of the topography code.

ICD-10 and the second and third editions of ICD-O have a more detailed set of topography codes. The site covered by some groups of codes is considered to be a single organ for the purposes of defining multiple tumors.

Multifocal tumors – that is, discrete masses apparently not in continuity with other primary cancers originating in the same primary site or tissue, for example, bladder – are counted as a single cancer.

Skin cancer presents a special problem, as the same individual may have many such neoplasms over a lifetime. The IARC/IACR rules imply that only the first tumor of a defined histological type, anywhere on the skin, is counted as an incident cancer, unless, for example, one primary was a malignant melanoma and the other a basal cell carcinoma.

Rule 3 above does not apply in 2 circumstances:

(1) For systemic or multicentric cancers potentially involving many discrete organs, some histological groups are handled as a class (e.g. leukemias, Kaposi sarcoma). They are counted only once in any individual.
(2) Other specific histologies are considered to be different for the purpose of defining multiple tumors. Thus, a tumor in the same organ with a different histology from the first primary is counted as a new tumor.

Synchronous primary cancers occur at or nearly at the same time, whereas metachronous neoplasms are separated by some defined time period [9]. Establishing the precise time period is one element of variability among cancer registries, making comparisons difficult. Driven by organizations such as SEER, the standard of 2 months or less for calling the cancer synchronous appears to be well accepted, but the cutoff for establishing whether or not cancers are indeed synchronous has ranged from as high as 1 year to as low as 1 month.

Another factor to be considered is the elapsed time from SPC initiation until the cancer is well enough established to diagnose. Thus, one cannot properly assign 'blame' for the second cancer to the treatment of the first cancer if the surveillance interval is too short to allow the SPC to develop. Carcinogenesis takes time, at least it appears to in all experimental situations.

The framework we have outlined so far allows us to define SPC with a degree of precision and in a manner consistent with at least some mainstream research practice. In short, SPCs are those MPCs that occur at least 2 months after the initial cancer. SPCs are, by definition, metachronous neoplasms [10]. Rigorously adopting this approach to understanding SPC has allowed certain authorities to then reserve MPCs for different neoplasms that happen *simultaneously* [11]. This would establish the

Box B: Selected SEER Rules for MPCs [20]

Rule 3a: Simultaneous multiple lesions of the same histological type within the same site (that is, multifocal tumors in a single organ or site) are a single primary. If 1 lesion has a behavior code of in situ /2 and the other lesion has a behavior code of malignant /3, this is a single primary whose behavior is malignant /3.

Example 1: At nephrectomy, 2 separate, distinct foci of renal cell carcinoma were found in the specimen, in addition to the 3.5-cm primary renal cell carcinoma. Abstract as a single primary.

Example 2: At mastectomy for removal of a 2-cm invasive ductal carcinoma, an additional 5-cm area of intraductal carcinoma was noted. Abstract as 1 invasive primary.

Rule 3b: If a new cancer of the same histology as an earlier one is diagnosed in the same site within 2 months, this is a single primary cancer.

Example: Adenocarcinoma in adenomatous polyp (8210) in sigmoid colon removed by polypectomy in December 2004. At segmental resection in January 2005, an adenocarcinoma in a tubular adenoma (8210) adjacent to the previous polypectomy site was removed. Count as 1 primary.

Rule 4: If both sides of a paired organ are involved with the same histological type within 2 months of the initial diagnosis,

(a) it is 1 primary if the physician states the tumor in 1 organ is metastatic from the other;
  (i) code the laterality to the side in which the primary originated;
  (ii) code the laterality as 4 if it is unknown in which side the primary originated;
(b) code as multiple primaries if the physician states these are independent primaries or when there is no physician statement that one is metastatic from the other.

Exception 1: Simultaneous bilateral involvement of the ovaries with the same histology is 1 primary and laterality is coded as 4 when it is unknown which ovary was the original site.

Exception 2: Bilateral retinoblastomas are a single primary with laterality of 4.

Exception 3: Bilateral Wilms tumors are always a single primary with laterality of 4.

Rule 5: If a tumor with the same histology is identified in the same site at least 2 months after the initial/original diagnosis (metachronous), it is a separate primary.

Exception 1: It is a single primary only when the physician documents that the initial/original tumor gave rise to the later tumor.

Example 1: Infiltrating duct carcinoma of the upper outer quadrant of the right breast diagnosed in March 2004 and treated with lumpectomy. Previously unidentified mass in left inner quadrant right breast noted in July 2004 mammogram. This was removed and found to be infiltrating ductal carcinoma. Abstract the case as 2 primaries.

Example 2: During the workup for a squamous cell carcinoma of the vocal cord, a second squamous cell carcinoma was discovered in the tonsillar fossa. Abstract as 2 primaries.

second primary and multiple primary as exclusive categories. We will not in fact follow the latter suggestion, but rather continue to use MPC to cover all cases involving a plurality of cancers arising independently of one another, *regardless of timing*.

To sum up, we are defining SPC as a neoplasm that arises independently in a new site or tissue and *subsequent* to the initial cancer, with the intervening period being at least 2 months [12].

Thus, SPCs are properly a *subset* of MPC. This is reflected in the adjoining semantic diagram we devised to capture the variety of plural cancers, mapped against the axes of time and space. The dotted line acknowledges that there is still some debate in the literature about how to classify and label subsequent cancers in a new site or tissue that arise prior to the 2-month point (fig. 2).

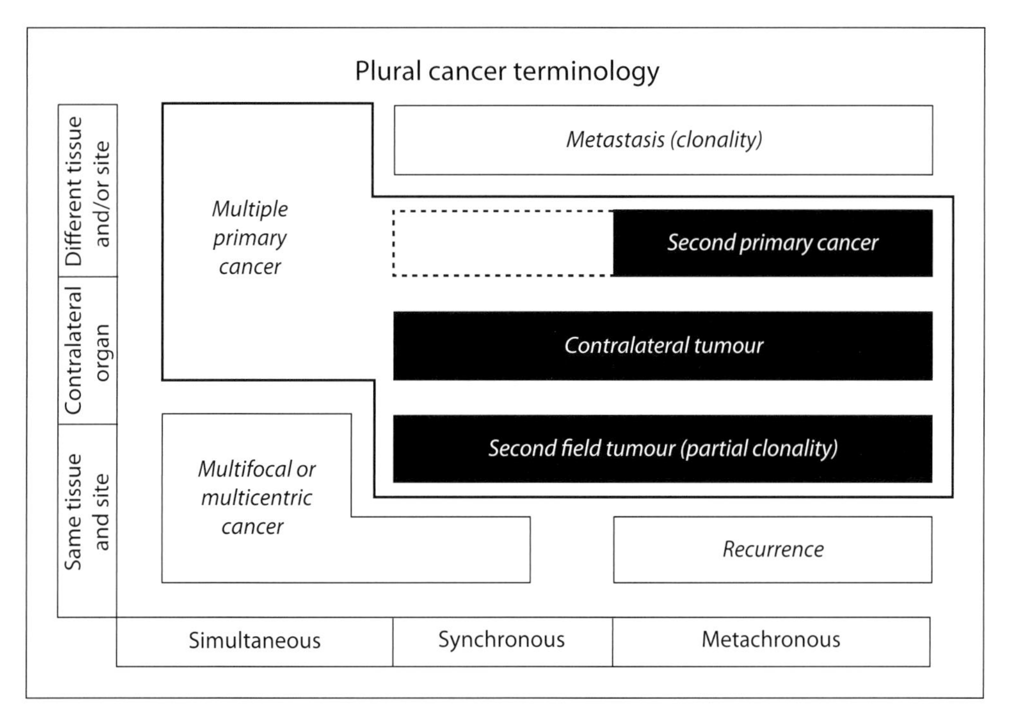

Fig. 2. Plural cancer terminology.

An immediate question arises around the epidemiological significance of the various plural cancer distinctions: by limiting the focus to metachronous cancers, how many synchronous conditions get removed from the statistics, and with what impact? The population level implications of our agreed definition of SPC can be quite profound. For example, adjustment of timing cutoff affects whether or not an excess risk is statistically significant, and, since prevention resources are driven by significance, it can also affect whether or not a prevention program is even developed.

The consequences of our proposed definition vary from site to site. In the case of head and neck cancers, SPC becomes distinguished from the sort of multiple neoplasms that are common in the mucosa of that region. There is sufficient clonality between such cancers to suggest that they are not quite 'new'. But at the same time, they are usually not classic metastases. As a consequence, researchers have posited theories of cancer spread within mucosal epithelium that occupy new definitional ground, leading to a category of cancers known as second field tumors. The same is true for cancers of the skin caused by exposure to UV light. We will return briefly to this lively topic of research later in the monograph. For now, it will suffice to point out that our 'tight' definition of SPC limits the official registry totals for the category.

It is important to qualify the application of the definition in terms of our literature review and synthesis. Because the work on the broad category of multiple cancers has been proceeding for over 100 years [13] under a wide range of terminology and definitions, we will be accessing studies that are not always as clear and precise as we might like with respect to terms such as multiple primary or second primary. We will gather data where we can, acknowledging that the analysis and conclusions may only approximate the 'true' results for the population. To put it differently, while cancer registries and related research are being steadily improved and coordinated, we must recognize that the past reality has created a mixed bag of results, and that the present improvement is at best a work in progress.

Finally, we note in passing that, even when some researchers are more liberal and apply the label 'second (primary) cancer' to both synchronous and metachronous types (see the dotted line in the chart above), they usually note that it is really the latter type that is of critical interest [9]. The practical reason for this is obvious: only a scenario involving metachronous cancers allows any realistic possibility of intervening to prevent the second cancer from developing or of detecting and treating it early. In the case of a synchronous cancer, it is simply too late to think of prevention. Thus, our tight definition of SPC certainly has operational utility from the point of view of developing prevention programs.

Synonyms for SPC

Having established the definitional boundaries of SPC, we still need to acknowledge the wide range of synonyms that intersects with the central concept. The simplest variation is the label 'second cancer' (where the idea of primary is assumed). Basically, the bulk of synonyms found in the literature relate to 1 of 2 variations: either the qualifier 'second' or 'second primary' is replaced with a term highlighting that the cancer is a side effect of therapy for the initial tumor, or an equivalent term for cancer is employed. This leads to what amounts to a synonym generator:

<table>
<tr><td colspan="2">second primary
second
second malignant [14]</td><td rowspan="2">cancer
malignancy
neoplasm
tumor</td></tr>
<tr><td>treatment
therapy</td><td>-associated
-related</td></tr>
</table>

Mixing and matching the possibilities creates more than 2 dozen different permutations, from second primary tumor to second malignant neoplasm to

Table 1. SPC literature by title vocabulary (published studies in Medline over 25 years)

	SPC(s)	Second primary neoplasm(s)	Second primary tumor(s)	Second primary malignancy(ies)	**Second primary [...] total**	Second cancer(s)
1981–1985	9	3	3	7	**22**	29
1986–1990	13	5	16	7	**41**	17
1991–1995	27	7	28	13	**75**	37
1996–2000	32	10	28	15	**85**	34
2001–2005	34	7	36	15	**92**	31
25-year total	115	32	111	57	**315**	148
	MPC(s)	Multiple primary neoplasm(s)	Multiple primary tumor(s)	Multiple primary malignancy(ies)	**Multiple primary [...] total**	Multiple cancer(s)
1981–1985	46	11	15	10	**82**	23
1986–1990	47	15	17	9	**88**	21
1991–1995	26	6	16	6	**54**	15
1996–2000	41	9	13	4	**67**	13
2001–2005	29	5	15	19	**68**	29
25-year total	189	46	76	48	**359**	101

therapy-associated malignancy, and so on. One caution is important: as a therapy-associated etiology represents only 1 of the possible causation pathways for SPC, it does not technically constitute a synonym but rather the marker of an important subset of the whole class. Specific therapies can be incorporated into an even narrower label, for example, radiation induced, alkylating agent mediated or cyclophosphamide caused. We note in passing that the term radiation induced is ambiguous, since it can refer to various sorts of environmental radiation (such as household radon, occupational exposure or diagnostic X-rays) that are not exclusively related to SPC.

It would be useful to know how the terminology is distributed in the literature. We conducted a survey of Medline in 5-year blocks over the last quarter century, which was based on a crude search of how often the indicated term appeared in its entirety as part of the title of a study. While this hardly exhausts the literature on SPC, nor even the use of the key terms, it does provide an impression of volume and trend in vocabulary choices. For comparison, we also tracked the usage of MPC and its main variations (table 1).

Table 2. Research published since 1981

	All terms
1981–1985	156
1986–1990	167
1991–1995	181
1996–2000	199
2001–2005	220
25-year total	**923**

The variety in usage is certainly confirmed, albeit within a general landscape where the 2 terms SPC and MPC dominate, and 'second primary tumor' is mounting a clear and growing challenge.

Three other observations may be offered:

(1) Adding the instances of 'second cancer' and 'multiple cancer' (that is, the last column), there is a remarkable balance in the total usage of 'second' and 'multiple' over 25 years (463 vs. 460).

(2) One could have guessed that, after the publication in 1999 of the seminal textbook entitled *Multiple Primary Cancer*s [15], MPC would begin to dominate the terminology in the 2000s. But the opposite trend appears to be occurring, that is, the slow, steady rise in popularity of 'second primary' (and its variants) against an apparent decline (or at least steady state) in the frequency of 'multiple primary'. At the same time, the shorthand forms, 'second cancer' and 'multiple cancer', seem to be used more consistently across the years.

(3) No matter what labels are used, the overall volume of publishing is steadily increasing, as seen in the totals of table 2.

If only the terms discussed so far exhausted all the options in the literature! Two other common phrases for treatment sequelae overlap substantially with the topic of SPC, namely, 'late effects (of therapy)' and 'long-term complications' with a third, 'survivorship issues' increasingly being seen [16]. Of course, many health impacts other than new cancers are also included under these headings, which in turn become wrapped up with the bigger discussion about cancer survivorship.

Finally, there are several other terms for SPC that are found occasionally in published material, including 'subsequent', 'new', 'additional' and even 'double cancer'. Sometimes, the terms from our preceding list are combined with the novel ones mentioned here, such as 'subsequent malignant neoplasm' [17]. Once we even encountered the label 'primary multiple cancer' – designed to keep one vigilant and flexible in the literature search process. The same may be said for titles that thoroughly disguise the connection with our topic, at least from the perspective of an automatic search in Medline. An example of this literature review challenge is the article 'Roles of radiotherapy and smoking in lung cancer following Hodgkin's disease' [18].

The overall inventory we have provided only serves to underline the difficult task of controlling the vast and varied literature on the theme of SPC. The ultimate aim is not, of course, to elucidate terminology. Instead, it is to retrieve and summarize the information that might make a difference to people at risk, while not muddying the picture with tangential topics that do not appreciably advance the clinical and public health agenda related to SPC. There is simply too much at stake to risk unhelpful detours. Just how much is at stake will be the subject of our next chapter.

Notes and References

1 Another way of thinking about this is that a primary cancer is malignancy found in the site where the cancer began. A primary cancer is usually named after the organ in which it starts (for example, breast cancer).

2 Metastasis refers to the spread of cancer from its original site to other parts of the body, usually through the bloodstream or lymphatic system.

3 Sometimes the term topology is used for this idea.

4 IACR: International Rules for Multiple Primary Cancers. Lyon, IACR, 2004. http://www.iacr.com.fr/MPrules_july2004.pdf (accessed March 2006).

5 Note that multifocal cancer is defined as disease appearing in more than 1 place in the same tissue and organ. In breast cancer, for example, smaller cancer spots may occur in the same quadrant of the breast as the main tumor. A related term exists. If there are smaller cancer spots in other quadrants than the one containing the main tumor, it is referred to as a multicentric condition.

6 A special case involves the skin. Because of the large number of neoplasms that may develop in this organ over a person's lifetime, some registries only count the first incidence of a nonmelanoma skin cancer of whatever tissue type. This means that, in practice, basal cell and squamous cell carcinomas are combined under one heading. In some registries, basal cell carcinomas are not recorded at all. See Moloney FJ, Comber H, Conlon PJ, et al: The role of immunosuppression in the pathogenesis of basal cell carcinoma. Br J Dermatol 2006;154:790–791.

7 It must be recognized that all coding conventions are driven by our best current understanding of carcinogenesis. New research may change the criteria and related registration decisions, that is, whether or not a cancer counts as really new. Work is always underway on harmonizing existing approaches. At the present time, SEER departs from the protocols adopted by IACR, as well as from other national systems (including the one used in Canada).

8 IACR: Recommendation for Coding Multiple Primaries. Lyon, IACR, 2000. www.encr.com.fr/multpeng.pdf (accessed March 2006).

9 Howe HL (ed): A Review of the Definition for Multiple Primary Cancers in the United States. Workshop Proceedings From December 4–6, 2002, in Princeton, New Jersey. Springfield, North American Association of Central Cancer Registries, 2003. Available at www. naaccr.org/filesystem/pdf/ PDF %20Multiple%20Primary%20Review%20FINAL%2005–13–03.pdf (accessed March 2006).

10 Dong C, Hemminki K: Second primary neoplasms in 633,964 cancer patients in Sweden, 1958–1996. Int J Cancer 2001;93:155–161.

11 Simultaneous primary cancers are in effect a subset of the synchronous category.

12 It should be acknowledged that this interval is often well exceeded. SPC of interest to epidemiologists can develop years rather than months after remission of the initial cancer. For instance, researchers are very concerned about cancers that emerge 2–3 decades later, often as a result of the therapy applied during the first malignancy.

13 Jakubowska D, Sielanczyk A, Kubacka M, et al: Multiple primary neoplasms in a century of research. Pol Arch Med Wewn 1999;101:65–67.

14 Obviously the qualifier 'malignant' would not be used with 'malignancy' from the final column.

15 Neugut AI, Meadows AT, Robinson E (eds): Multiple Primary Cancers. Philadelphia, Lippincott Williams & Wilkins, 1999.
16 Much less common is the term 'late complications'.
17 Sankila R, Pukkala E, Teppo L: Risk of subsequent malignant neoplasms among 470,000 cancer patients in Finland, 1953–1991. Int J Cancer 1995;60: 464–470.
18 van Leeuwen FE, Klokman WJ, Stovall M, et al: Roles of radiotherapy and smoking in lung cancer following Hodgkin's disease. J Natl Cancer Inst 1995; 87:1530–1537.
19 Available at http://www.iacr.com.fr/multprim.pdf (accessed June 2006).
20 Available at http://seer.cancer.gov/manuals/SPM 2004_ replace_04052005.pdf (accessed June 2006).

Krueger H, McLean D, Williams D: The Prevention of Second Primary Cancers.
Prog Exp Tumor Res. Basel, Karger, 2008, vol 40, pp 17–24

3

Importance of SPC

Cases involving SPC have become increasingly important in the last 25 years. Partly this reflects the fact that they now comprise the sixth most common category of malignancy after skin, colorectal, lung, breast and prostate cancers [1]. Beyond this general sense of priority, the research interest in SPC has been sharpened for 3 compelling reasons:

- The potential for reducing risk of SPC through modifications of host behavior (such as smoking and sexual health), control of passive environmental exposures or adjustments in medical therapy.
- The fact that epidemiologic data can guide surveillance priorities among patients particularly at risk for SPC. The goal in such situations is early detection and intervention.
- The general insights about carcinogenesis that may be learned from the mechanisms behind SPC, especially related to inherent genetic susceptibility [2–5].

In terms of the first rationale, it is fair to ask: what are the true population health implications of SPC? In other words, what urgency should be attached to any program of risk factor reduction? One route of assessment involves large epidemiologic studies of first primary cancer survivors. The results have shown for the most part only a modest increase in the risk of SPC for all survivors of all cancers, as seen in table 3 [6].

Although the statistical power of, for example, the large Swedish sample is compelling, even its results cannot overcome the general impression that the excess risk of SPC across the entire population of cancer survivors is not that high. One finding reflected in the table is the apparent higher risk of SPC for females compared to males. The gender difference is likely due to second cancers of the breast and gynecologic organs [7]. This result should not obscure the main point: although all studies demonstrated a SIR of more than 1.0, the overall excess is modest and does not raise a loud alarm about SPC. However, patients, clinicians and population health leaders rarely deal with all cancers as an aggregate topic. Instead, they deal with specific malignancies or classes of malignancies, and thus are usually looking for more focused information. The limited usefulness of studies that offer aggregate data across

Table 3. Excess risk of SPC following all first primaries

Country	Sample period	Sample size	SIR	95% CI
US (1985) [7]	1935–1982	~254,000	all: 1.23 male: 1.19 females: 1.42	1.21–1.25 $p < 0.05$ $p < 0.05$
Denmark (1985) [8]	1943–1980	~380,000	all: 1.06 [9] male: 1.03 females: 1.08	1.04–1.09
Switzerland (1993) [10]	1974–1989	~34,600	1.20 for both males and females	$p < 0.001$
Finland (1995) [11]	1953–1991	~470,000	all: 1.12 males: 1.00 females: 1.25	1.10–1.13 0.98–1.01 1.23–1.27
Sweden (2001) [12]	1958–1996	~634,000	males: 1.3 females: 1.6	1.2–1.3 1.5–1.6
Italy (2001) [13]	1976–1995	~240,000	1.08	1.05–1.12

CI = Confidence interval.

all first primaries may account for the scarcity of such broad-based assessments since 2001.

To sum up, if the aggregate table presented earlier (table 3) contained all the information we had, there might be limited concern about SPC. The picture already begins to refocus, though, when age at diagnosis is considered. This was anticipated in the Finnish study noted in table 3, where patients younger than 50 years of age demonstrated a significant SIR of 1.7 for SPC. To recap: SIR is defined as the ratio of observed cancer incidence (among cancer survivors) to expected occurrences (in a general population) [14]. A SIR of 1.7 means that there is a 70% increase in cancer risk – not a trivial amount.

The results for childhood cancer survivors may be even more dramatic. For example, the risk of thyroid cancer in childhood survivors of Hodgkin's disease is more than 13 times, or 1,300%, more than normal. In this light, the topic of SPC is of particular relevance for those working with children and adolescents. We will expand on this area in the balance of this chapter, and again at the end of the monograph. What will become clear is that, apart from any general considerations of burden, data on specific SPC risks in specific cohorts will always be vital to know.

Pediatric Implications

SPCs are especially important in pediatric oncology, not because they usually develop in childhood but because so many cases have been linked to the treatments used to fight the original primary in children and adolescents. Thus, even though it may be adult survivors of childhood cancer who are afflicted by the various SPCs, the preventive measures necessarily begin in the context of pediatric care. The one exception to this pattern is any tumor that develops in children as a result of intrauterine radiation exposure related to treatment of cancer in a pregnant mother. Although such cancers are 'first primaries' for the child, they could be considered as effects following therapy and thus a logical parallel to SPC. The preventive interventions of interest in such cases obviously begin with the cancer care received by the mother.

Childhood cancer is uncommon everywhere in the world, with an age-standardized incidence between 7 and 16 per 100,000 children up to age 14 [15]. Logically, SPC following such cancers cannot occur too often across the whole population (a proportion of a small total is always going to be small). But the concern goes far beyond objective disease burden and costs. It is hard to quantify the psychological impact of developing a new cancer after surviving the already emotional experience of a childhood cancer. Even a few such cases within a local community can be devastating for patients and their family and friends. By comparison, research has shown that a high degree of distress is even caused when participants in epidemiological studies learn that there are elevated risks for getting such tumors [16]. SPC is a sensitive and emotional topic, naturally made worse when it actually occurs. Exacerbating any immediate psychological effect is the fact that the morbidity and mortality attached to certain types of SPC is very high.

As a result of these and other issues, there has been intense interest in developing preventive measures to interrupt the development of SPCs in survivors of pediatric cancer.

As we indicated in the opening chapter, the concern about SPC in childhood cancer survivors is a by-product of medical success. If the people involved had not survived their pediatric cancer in the first place, then there would be no treatment-related consequences to either prevent or manage. This ironic reality inspires commentaries such as a recent editorial entitled 'Long-term sequelae after cancer therapy – a necessary consequence of success?' [17]

The survival rate related to most pediatric cancers has been steadily rising. In the developed world, about 75% of children diagnosed with cancer survive at least 5 years, and most are cured. Mortality beyond 5 years is usually related to recurrent tumors, which account for almost three quarters of late deaths [18]. The next most serious causes of mortality are cardiac or pulmonary complications, with SPCs positioned in third spot (or perhaps tied for second) [19]. For instance, a British study of 4,082 childhood cancer survivors surviving at least 5 years found that, of the 749 deaths in the following 15 years, 61 (8%) were attributable to SPC [20].

The Childhood Cancer Survivor Study (CCSS) has yielded important information about the impact of SPC: deaths caused by such malignancies are 19 times more frequent in cancer survivors than when the cancer occurs in the general population. Overall, the CCSS has found SPC to be the second or third most common cause of death in childhood cancer survivors [21].

Radiation and certain chemotherapies used to treat first primaries in children have been implicated in a higher risk of SPC. It remains to be seen just what proportion of SPC following childhood cancer is really an alternate way of talking about iatrogenic effects related to treatment. In other words, is the phenomenon mainly a by-product of medical care rather than any cause specific to the patient's biology or behavior? The answer to this question clearly would shape an appropriate clinical or public health response.

A goal in caring for pediatric cancer patients and their families is to follow up the positive experience of surviving cancer with accurate information about risks of SPC. The objective is to enhance surveillance and achieve early diagnosis/intervention where possible. Even better, if there are modifiable risks (such as smoking) related to SPC development, preventive steps can be encouraged and supported among cancer survivors.

As already suggested, a fundamental clinical objective would be to ensure that medical care related to the first cancer is not unnecessarily contributing to the incidence of SPC. As will be seen in the case of adult-onset cancers, treatment modalities in childhood cancer have long been implicated in the etiology of subsequent tumors. The key question becomes: are there modified or alternate therapies that will still be effective in controlling pediatric cancer without causing as many adverse effects, including an excess risk of SPC? This same concern is reflected in the drive to reduce diagnostic radiation exposures to as low a level as reasonably achievable (generating the acronym ALARA).

Burden of Pediatric SPC

A comprehensive assessment of the problem of SPC following childhood cancer must consider and correlate the following variables:

- type of childhood cancer
- age at treatment
- type, intensity and duration of treatment
- duration of and attained age at follow-up
- environmental or genetic factors that increase susceptibility to SPC.

Currently, 2 large continuing studies are examining SPC and other adverse health outcomes following childhood cancer: the CCSS (established in 1992 among 25 clinical centers in the US and Canada) [22] and the British CCSS (launched in 1998). Other large national and regional studies are also found in the literature, including the ones based in the US (Late Effects Study Group) and in the Nordic countries [23]. The most recent report of this sort was published in 2007, based on US SEER data [24]. Comparing the results of these various studies is illuminating (table 4) [25].

Table 4. Excess risk of SPC following pediatric first primaries

Country	Sample size	Diagnosis before age	Cumulative risk	Excess risk over general population (SIR)
Britain	10,106	15	4.0% (25)	6.0
Britain [26]	16,541 [27]	15	4.2% (25)	6.2
Nordic countries	30,880	20	2.6% (20)	3.6
US/Canada	13,581 [28]	21	3.2% (20)	6.4
US/Canada [29]	13,136	21		4.0
Canada (BC) [30]	2,322	20		5.0 [31]
US [24]	25,965	18		5.9

Figures in parentheses are the years of follow-up.

In a sense, the last column in this table is the most important. While cumulative risks for SPC following childhood cancer as high as 12% or even 20% have been recorded, the vital task is always to determine the excess risk attributable to surviving a first primary cancer. Although there is remarkable consistency across the results shown in the table, we should note that other research has indicated even higher relative risks for SPC, up to 15-fold [32]. Therefore, the excess risk in the last column may represent a conservative result.

The trend line is alarming. According to 1 study, there is no evidence that the risk of SPC is being reduced by newer treatment protocols or other factorial changes [33]. In fact, there is a concern that excess risk for some forms of SPC has actually been increasing for patients diagnosed more recently – a phenomenon that may be related to more intensive therapy [26, 34].

Looking more closely at the range of first primaries, CCSS concluded that there was 'a statistically significant excess' of SPC following any childhood malignancy [35]. The details vary according to the specific first cancer. There are 4 pediatric cancers associated with SPC that have received a lot of attention [34]:

(1) Hodgkin's disease
(2) acute lymphocytic leukemia [36]
(3) Wilms tumor of the kidney
(4) retinoblastoma of the eye.

For instance, a review of the research studies concerning pediatric Hodgkin's disease generated the following summary of SPC risk (table 5) [37]. The last column in this table introduces a new statistic, the absolute excess risk (AER). What this means is that up to 7 excess cases of subsequent cancer will be expected per 1,000 child survivors of Hodgkin's disease over the course of 1 year; as with SIRs, the excess is measured against the expected number of cases in the general population. The AER is

Table 5. Excess risk of SPC following pediatric Hodgkin's disease

Lead researcher	Year	Sample size	SIR	95% CI	AER (per 1,000 person years)
Bassal [38]	2006	1,927	3.40	2.10–5.40	
Bhatia [40]	2003	1,380	18.50	15.60–21.70	6.50
Neglia [35]	2001	1,815	9.70	8.05–11.59	5.13
Metayer [37]	2000	5,925	7.70	6.60–8.80	2.70–3.60
Green [37]	2000	182	males: 9.39 females: 10.16	4.05–18.49 5.56–17.05	
Van Leeuwen [37]	2000	1,253	7.00	5.90–8.30	7.23

CI = Confidence interval; AER = absolute excess risk.

becoming more popular as a reported statistic, as it gives an immediate sense of the absolute health burden represented by a SPC.

Beyond the 4 pediatric malignancies listed above, other first primary cancers in childhood that have significant association with SPC include bone malignancies (notably Ewing's sarcoma), brain and central nervous system tumors, neuroblastoma and soft tissue sarcomas [39].

It is also important to be aware of the most frequent cancers found in pediatric cancer survivors. Two major types of SPC following pediatric first primaries are chemotherapy-related acute nonlymphocytic leukemia (or its precursor, myelodysplastic syndrome) and radiation-associated solid (nonhematopoietic) tumors [40, 41].

The general rule of thumb for second solid tumors is that they are often radiation associated and expected to develop late. This is not the case for all SPC. The generally high and early (within 10 years) risk for some forms of SPC is the motivation behind intensive surveillance of childhood cancer survivors from the start of the follow-up period. In short, there is no room for complacency based on a presumed long latency period for any new cancer. We will cover further details concerning epidemiology and prevention of SPC related to specific childhood cancers later in the monograph (see chapter 14, pp 122–134).

A related topic involves the 'second generation' effect. This refers to the fact that children born to childhood cancer survivors also require heightened surveillance for the occurrence of cancer and other adverse effects. A parallel phenomenon is the fact that siblings of those who contract certain types of cancer (including SPC) also experience an elevated risk of cancer development. This occurs when the underlying cause of cancer has a genetic component that is inherent in relatives and inheritable by offspring. As we learn more about the specific gene abnormalities that lead to some cancers, and as tests for such genes become available and cost-effective, such surveillance will be targetable to those at specific risk [42].

To sum up, we must continue to monitor the outcome data related to childhood cancer, especially in light of changing treatment protocols [43]. While it is true that, 'in comparison with almost certain death from untreated childhood cancer, the absolute risks of [SPC] experienced by survivors are small' [26], it is still important to reduce risks wherever possible, or at least to guard against any trend towards increased risk. The challenge for pediatric oncologists is always 'to develop minimally toxic therapy strategies, while retaining maximum effectiveness regarding survival and quality of life' [41].

Notes and References

1 Rheingold SR, Neugut AI, Meadows AT: Secondary cancers: incidence, risk factors and management; in Bast RC, Kufe DW, Pollock RE, et al (eds): Cancer Medicine. Hamilton, B.C. Decker, 2000, pp 2399–2406.

2 Hart P: The role of the retinoblastoma gene in tumour pathogenesis. Clin Oncol 1992;4:125–129.

3 Kaye FJ, Harbour JW: For whom the bell tolls: susceptibility to common adult cancers in retinoblastoma survivors. J Natl Cancer Inst 2004;96:342–343.

4 Hemminki K, Boffetta P: Multiple primary cancers as clues to environmental and heritable causes of cancer and mechanisms of carcinogenesis. IARC Sci Publ 2004;157:289–297.

5 Engeland A, Bjorge T, Haldorsen T, et al: Use of multiple primary cancers to indicate associations between smoking and cancer incidence: an analysis of 500,000 cancer cases diagnosed in Norway during 1953–93. Int J Cancer 1997;70:401–407.

6 Some data are summarized in Bhatia S, Sklar C: Second cancers in survivors of childhood cancer. Nat Rev Cancer 2002;2:124–132.

7 Curtis RE, Boice JD Jr, Kleinerman RA, et al: Summary: multiple primary cancers in Connecticut, 1935–82. Natl Cancer Inst Monogr 1985;68:219–242.

8 Storm HH, Jensen OM, Ewertz M, et al: Summary: multiple primary cancers in Denmark, 1943–80. Natl Cancer Inst Monogr 1985;68:411–430.

9 Excluding the first 5 years of observation due to coding practices.

10 Levi F, Randimbison L, Te VC, et al: Multiple primary cancers in the Vaud Cancer Registry, Switzerland, 1974–89. Br J Cancer 1993;67:391–395.

11 Sankila R, Pukkala E, Teppo L: Risk of subsequent malignant neoplasms among 470,000 cancer patients in Finland, 1953–1991. Int J Cancer 1995;60: 464–470.

12 Dong C, Hemminki K: Second primary neoplasms in 633,964 cancer patients in Sweden, 1958–1996. Int J Cancer 2001;93:155–161.

13 Crocetti E, Buiatti E, Falini P: Multiple primary cancer incidence in Italy. Eur J Cancer 2001;37: 2449–2456.

14 Thus, it is sometimes abbreviated in reports as O/E.

15 Stiller CA: Epidemiology and genetics of childhood cancer. Oncogene 2004;23:6429–6444.

16 Schulz CJ, Riddle MP, Valdimirsdottir HB, et al: Impact on survivors of retinoblastoma when informed of study results on risk of second cancers. Med Pediatr Oncol 2003;41:36–43.

17 Glimelius B: Long-term sequelae after cancer therapy – a necessary consequence of success? Acta Oncol 2004;43:132–133.

18 Robertson CM, Hawkins MM, Kingston JE: Late deaths and survival after childhood cancer: implications for cure. BMJ 1994;309:162–166.

19 Hawkins MM: Long-term survivors of childhood cancers: what knowledge have we gained? Nat Clin Pract 2004;1:26–31.

20 Hawkins MM, Kingston JE, Kinnier Wilson LM: Late deaths after treatment for childhood cancer. Arch Dis Child 1990;65:1356–1363.

21 Mertens AC, Yaui Y, Neglia JP, et al: Late mortality experience in five-year survivors of childhood and adolescent cancer: the Childhood Cancer Survivor Study. J Clin Oncol 2001;19:3163–3172.

22 Robison LL, Mertens AC, Boice JD, et al: Study design and cohort characteristics of the Childhood Cancer Survivor Study: a multi-institutional collaborative project. Med Pediatr Oncol 2002;38:229–239.

23 Olsen JH, Garwicz S, Hertz H, et al: Second malignant neoplasms after cancer in childhood or adolescence. Nordic Society of Paediatric Haematology and Oncology Association of the Nordic Cancer Registries. BMJ 1993;307:1030–1036.

24 Inskip PD, Curtis RE: New malignancies following childhood cancer in the United States, 1973–2002. Int J Cancer 2007;121:2233–2240.

25 Unless otherwise indicated, results in this table are adapted from Hawkins MM: Long-term survivors of childhood cancers: what knowledge have we gained? Nat Clin Pract 2004;1:26–31.

26 Jenkinson HC, Hawkins MM, Stiller CA, et al: Long-term population-based risks of second malignant neoplasms after childhood cancer in Britain. Br J Cancer 2004;91:1905–1910.

27 Cases of skin cancer excluded.

28 Cases of retinoblastoma excluded.

29 This represents the most recent and relevant update from the CCSS. It is limited to second primary carcinomas. See Bassal M, Mertens AC, Taylor L, et al: Risk of selected subsequent carcinomas in survivors of childhood cancer: a report from the Childhood Cancer Survivor Study. J Clin Oncol 2006;24:476–483.

30 MacArthur AC, Spinelli JJ, Rogers PC, et al: Risk of a second malignant neoplasm among 5-year survivors of cancer in childhood and adolescence in British Columbia, Canada. Pediatr Blood Cancer 2007;48: 453–459.

31 Nonmelanoma skin cancer excluded.

32 Westermeier T, Kaatsch P, Schoetzau A, et al: Multiple primary neoplasms in childhood: data from the German Children's Cancer Registry. Eur J Cancer 1998;34:687–693.

33 Hammal DM, Bell CL, Craft AW, et al: Second primary tumors in children and young adults in the North of England (1968–99). Pediatr Blood Cancer 2005;45:155–161.

34 Moppett J, Oakhill A, Duncan AW: Second malignancies in children: the usual suspects? Eur J Radiol 2001;37:235–248.

35 Neglia JP, Friedman DL, Yasui Y, et al: Second malignant neoplasms in five-year survivors of childhood cancer: childhood cancer survivor study. J Natl Cancer Inst 2001;93:618–629.

36 Another common name for this cancer is acute lymphoblastic leukemia.

37 The data in the table was adapted from in Lin HM, Teitell MA: Second malignancy after treatment of pediatric Hodgkin disease. J Pediatr Hematol Oncol 2005;27:28–36 and updated with more recent references as indicated.

38 This represents the most recent update of the CCSS and is limited to second primary carcinomas. See the next reference.

39 Bassal M, Mertens AC, Taylor L, et al: Risk of selected subsequent carcinomas in survivors of childhood cancer: a report from the Childhood Cancer Survivor Study. J Clin Oncol 2006;24:476–483.

40 Bhatia S: What is the risk of second malignant neoplasms after childhood cancer? Nat Clin Pract 2005; 2:182–183.

41 Klein G, Michaelis J, Spix C, et al: Second malignant neoplasms after treatment of childhood cancer. Eur J Cancer 2003;39:808–817.

42 Friedman DL, Kadan-Lottick NS, Whitton J: Increased risk of cancer among siblings of long-term childhood cancer survivors: a report from the Childhood Cancer Survivor Study. Cancer Epidemiol Biomarkers Prev 2005;14:1922–1927.

43 Meadows AT: Second tumours. Eur J Cancer 2001; 37:2074–2079; discussion 2079–2081.

Krueger H, McLean D, Williams D: The Prevention of Second Primary Cancers.
Prog Exp Tumor Res. Basel, Karger, 2008, vol 40, pp 25–31

4

Framework and Methodology

In assembling the SPC story from the literature, it was important to acknowledge some of the limitations attached to the data. We discuss the relevant challenges in this chapter, providing an overview of our review strategy.

Diagnostic and Epidemiologic Challenges

Pediatric oncology alone is beset by specific research issues. First, there is the technical question about what constitutes childhood or, more specifically, adolescence. The selected age cutoffs used to shape statistical data are important from a biological point of view. For example, there is concern about radiation to the chest in girls during puberty, when cells in the breast are in a high mitotic state, and thus susceptible to mutations and increased rates of cancer. Will the organization of a database help to reveal such associations? As well, when various pediatric registries are built around different cutoffs (age 15, 16 or even later) comparison and meta-analysis of data are more difficult. With this scenario, the breast cancer risk 'carried' by younger cancer survivors could be missed, as could other age-specific pockets of risk.

A second challenge involves the long latency period before SPC develops – as long as 40 years [1]. It is sobering to realize that females diagnosed with cancer at age 5–20 would only be age 25–40 after 20 years of follow-up – still relatively young for developing breast cancer. Thus, the full effects of any contemporary advances in childhood cancer therapy may not yet have been revealed.

Third, there are complex issues related to age at follow-up. An important application of this again involves breast cancer following childhood cancer. Standard analyses have sometimes failed to take into consideration the natural rise of breast cancer risk with age [2]. The background population risk for all cancers after 45 years of follow-up is almost 6% [3].

Widening the discussion to include adults, another factor that needs to be controlled is the difference in treatment protocols between countries, and the changes in standard therapy or 'usual care' over time.

There are a number of ways crude data can be adjusted beyond the category of treatment variables. When comparing 2 studies, a relevant question is: have the adjustments been made in a consistent way? And what if the figures are not adjusted at all? Evaluating trends and associations based only on crude data can be problematic.

Finally, because of the complex, multifactorial etiology and the rarity of some types of SPC, large-scale epidemiologic investigations are required [4]. The use of population-wide registries based on standardized coding rules is generally considered to be superior to patient series developed out of cancer follow-up clinics (where the resulting cohorts may be unrepresentative) [5].

Issues of accuracy and reliability have an impact on the key metric we report in this monograph, namely, the SIR. Being a ratio, the SIR will only be as solid as the quality of the numerator and denominator. This means deriving good figures for the expected number of cancer cases in a general population as well as for the observed cancers following a first primary. When the sample is modest or the observed cases are limited, it is not appropriate to lean too heavily on any conclusions. There is the possibility of what is known as small number error. For example, if only 10 people in a registry develop a certain SPC, then any 'random variation' or under-reporting bias (even involving only a small number of cases) will create a huge proportional impact.

Parameters of the Search

The key text in this area of cancer research and treatment dates from 1999. *Multiple Primary Cancers*, edited by Neugat and colleagues, consisted of a series of detailed review articles written by global experts, covering the important data available up to about 10 years ago [6]. Thus, we immediately had the first criteria for our literature review: it would be important to find any research of major consequence published since 1997. The main data of interest comprised the epidemiology of SPC and any risk factors and prevention approaches. Experimental evidence on the topic of preventing SPC is usually very limited.

We suggested in chapter 2 (pp 7–16) that one of the greatest challenges involved with accessing Medline and other indexes is the fact that the terms related to SPC are many and varied. We ultimately searched using a couple of a dozen different phrases in order to capture as many review articles and key studies as possible.

Beyond the issue of using the appropriate key terms, it is important to acknowledge that the topic of SCP is covered from a number of different perspectives. There are at least 7 research categories:

(1) SPC in general
(2) SPC following a special category of first primaries, such as pediatric cancers
(3) SPC as one aspect of a late effect after cancer treatment (usually administered in childhood)

Table 6. Sample headings for comprehensive SIR data

SPC	Overall SIR	Years of follow-up: SIR			
		<1 year	1–4 years	5–9 years	≥10 years

(4) all or specific SPC following a specific first primary (or following a category of tumors, such as head and neck cancer or hematologic malignancies)
(5) a particular SPC following all types of first primaries
(6) SPC following certain cancer therapies (sometimes focusing on the treatment effects related to a specific therapy for a specific first primary)
(7) prevention of SPC, either specific or general.

There has been a significant volume of publishing over the last decade in all areas listed, with the exception of the last category. We will derive the epidemiology mostly from the direct data contained in the middle research category, that is, SIR results for all SPCs following each first primary. Our first interest is any evidence of elevated risk of cancer following a first primary; this eliminates the small body of literature that reports incidence of SPC but does not calculate the excess incidence [7].

Strategy of the Review and Synthesis

To generate the data concerning SPC risk, we will consult either a recent review (if it provides a meta-analysis) or an 'index' study chosen according to the following criteria: it must be relatively recent (generally published since the comprehensive textbook from 1999, *Multiple Primary Cancers*) and use a sizeable sample, preferably one derived from a population-wide cohort rather than a clinical series.

The superstructure of our review will be a series of tables that succinctly lay out the risk of key SPCs following a specified first primary. The fullest version of a table will include information gathered in different follow-up periods, as shown in table 6. Sometimes, either the overall SIR or the time period data were not provided in the index study. Occasionally, the available research allowed us to stratify by gender.

Generally, we will only present the SIR data that are statistically significant [8]. Given this basic criterion concerning the significance of the figures, we sometimes elect to omit the 95% confidence intervals (CI) in order to keep the tables streamlined. The strategy of focusing on significant data creates a new convention, one that avoids the usual comprehensive (and often bewildering) presentation of all results, whether the SIRs are significant or not. Our approach seeks to highlight the instances of excess risk (and the rare cases of a protective effect) following the first primary [9].

Table 7. PYLL (British Columbia, Canada, 2003)

Cancer type	Number of deaths	Residual life expectancy	PYLL	% of total PYLL
All adult cancers	7,875	14.7	115,786	100.0
Lung	2,030	14.7	29,742	25.7
Colorectal	954	13.5	12,912	11.2
Breast	588	18.8	11,064	9.6
Pancreas	454	14.3	6,471	5.6
Non-Hodgkin's lymphoma	320	14.6	4,673	4.0
Ovary	244	17.8	4,331	3.7
Brain	206	19.9	4,098	3.5
Prostate	430	8.4	3,613	3.1
Leukemia	259	13.4	3,461	3.0
Esophagus	224	14.8	3,312	2.9
Stomach	205	14.5	2,967	2.6
Kidney	169	14.7	2,479	2.1
Oral	142	17.1	2,426	2.1
Bladder	203	11.0	2,227	1.9
Melanoma, skin	114	17.6	2,008	1.7
Multiple myeloma	143	13.3	1,898	1.6
Cervix	51	25.9	1,320	1.1
Body of uterus	80	15.5	1,236	1.1
Larynx	40	15.0	602	0.5
Thyroid	20	16.5	330	0.3
Testis	8	32.5	260	0.2
Hodgkin's disease	8	15.7	126	0.1
All other cancers	983	14.5	14,230	12.3
Childhood cancers	29	66.3	1,923	

Adapted from Data for 2003 PYLL (www.bccancer.bc.ca).

As well as isolating significant data, we will organize the results according to the estimated impact of the SPC. In effect, we ask: how serious is it, from the point of view of morbidity and/or mortality, to actually develop the second malignancy? And how does this impact translate across a population? There are different ways to make such an assessment. As indicated earlier, we have chosen to use PYLL to calibrate the health consequences for a population. The ranking is specifically achieved by assessing the overall proportion of PYLL due to that cancer in British Columbia, Canada, according to mortality data from 2003 (table 7) [10]. British Columbia has a population of 4.4 million with an excellent population-based cancer registry. The grid will be appropriate for most developed jurisdictions, though any required adjustments can be easily made. In other words, a particular country or region may want to elevate the profile of a certain SPC of concern.

Demonstrating the implication of our grid, 25.7% of all PYLL due to cancers in British Columbia in 2003 were attributable to lung cancers (including first primaries, second primaries, etc.); this is the highest percentage of all cancers by a wide margin, meaning that any SPC of the lung will always appear first in any summary table in this monograph. The justification for this approach is as follows: as PYLL is a combination metric indicating something about both the volume of a disease and its prognosis, it serves as a good 'window' on the population impact of any SPC. In short, a cancer at a particular site with high PYLL may be considered to generate a larger absolute number of cases in the province, or a high mortality rate, or both. The potential population impact of second primary related to such a site follows accordingly. Of course, beyond the crude ranking this allows, we are especially interested in any SPC with a significant and substantial excess risk following a first primary. In other words, regardless of the order in the table, the size of the SIR must also be carefully assessed.

We will not be restricted to population-based priorities. The impact of SPC on an individual who has already survived a first primary is difficult to measure, but it certainly extends beyond bare statistics. This is especially true for someone who has experienced a pediatric cancer. So, our summary tables will sometimes leave behind the PYLL ranking system and report a SPC with a high mortality rate, that is, where it also demonstrates a high SIR. Prevention and surveillance related to such cancers conceivably ought to have some degree of priority in an overall program, given their devastating impact on patients and their families. An indication of the prognosis for cancers can be derived from survival rates. Table 8 indicates the proportion of individuals with various cancers that will survive at least 5 years [11].

The survival rates for pancreatic, liver, esophageal and lung cancers are dramatically low. This partly explains the placement of lung cancer first and pancreatic as well as esophageal cancer in the first half of the PYLL rankings in British Columbia (see above). Liver cancer, though not appearing in the PYLL rankings (due to its rarity), nevertheless deserves mention in our analysis whenever appropriate, given the gravity of developing that particular malignancy. The appropriateness of including liver cancer in our summaries depends, as always, on whether there is a significant and sizeable excess risk of its incidence following the first primary under consideration.

What We Left Out

This monograph, while extensive, is not exhaustive. A few other types of cancer could be drawn into the conversation, but will be bypassed in order to make sure the most important information does not get lost in the details. The omitted stories include first primaries where research has been modest and/or there is no compelling evidence of excess SPCs. Osteosarcoma and male breast cancer, among others, fit this category.

Another case of more modest interest would be brain and central nervous system malignancies. As table 9 shows, the indication of significant excess risk for all cancers

Table 8. Relative 5-year survival rate estimates

Cancer site	Survival rate (%)
Pancreas	4.0
Liver and intrahepatic bile duct	7.5
Esophagus	14.2
Lung and bronchus	15.0
Stomach	23.8
Multiple myeloma	29.5
Brain and other nervous system	32.0
Leukemias	42.5
Ovary	55.0
Oral cavity and pharynx	56.7
Non-Hodgkin's lymphoma	57.8
Colon	61.7
Kidney and renal pelvis	61.8
Rectum	62.6
Larynx	68.8
Cervix uteri	70.5
Urinary bladder	82.1
Corpus uteri and uterus, NOS	84.3
Hodgkin's disease	85.1
Breast	86.4
Melanomas	89.0
Testis	94.7
Thyroid	96.0
Prostate	98.8

NOS = Not otherwise specified. Adapted from Brenner et al. [11].

Table 9. SPC following cancer of the brain and central nervous system

SPC	Overall SIR
Brain and nervous system	5.89 (4.12–8.15)
Brain	4.85 (3.22–7.01)
Other central nervous system	23.60 (10.20–46.20)
Leukemia	2.63 (1.71–3.85)
Acute myeloid leukemia	4.08 (1.95–7.50)
Thyroid gland	2.70 (1.47–4.53)
Soft tissue sarcomas	4.64 (2.22–8.53)
Salivary glands	5.07 (1.63–11.80)
Bone	14.40 (7.43–25.20)
All cancers	**1.10 (1.00–1.21)**

Figures in parentheses are 95% CI. Adapted from Inskip [12].

is lacking, though there is evidence for higher incidence of leukemia as well as certain solid tumors, notably in the nervous system itself [12].

The limited research with respect to brain cancer as a first primary may reflect the situation seen in esophageal and liver cancer: the prognosis is so poor after the original malignancy that there is little opportunity for SPC development. This does not mean that SPC following brain cancer does not warrant further study and clinical focus. Those dealing with childhood brain tumors, while acknowledging the low absolute excess risk, would naturally call for a surveillance program, especially because the consequences of getting a SPC following pediatric brain cancer is particularly serious [13].

We will now turn to the major cancers with SPC implications. Each of the following chapters is organized around a first primary, or a well-established group of first primaries (for example, head and neck cancers). Finally, we will return to the topic of SPC following pediatric cancers.

Notes and References

1 Robison LL: Methodologic issues in the study of second malignant neoplasms and pregnancy outcomes. Med Pediatr Oncol 1996;1:41–44.
2 Yasui Y, Liu Y, Neglia JP, et al: A methodological issue in the analysis of second-primary cancer incidence in long-term survivors of childhood cancers. Am J Epidemiol 2003;158:1108–1113.
3 Moppett J, Oakhill A, Duncan AW: Second malignancies in children: the usual suspects? Eur J Radiol 2001;37:235–248.
4 Hawkins MM: Long-term survivors of childhood cancers: what knowledge have we gained? Nat Clin Pract 2004;1:26–31.
5 Westermeier T, Kaatsch P, Schoetzau A, et al: Multiple primary neoplasms in childhood: data from the German Children's Cancer Registry. Eur J Cancer 1998;34:687–693.
6 Neugut AI, Meadows AT, Robinson E (eds): Multiple Primary Cancers. Philadelphia, Lippincott Williams & Wilkins, 1999.
7 For example Caglar K, Varan A, Akyuz C, et al: Second neoplasms in pediatric patients treated for cancer: a center's 30-year experience. J Pediatr Hematol Oncol 2006;28:374–378.
8 On the occasions when we depart from this standard, we will note it explicitly.
9 Interested readers are referred to the original papers to fill in the nonsignificant blanks.
10 Data for 2003 PYLL (www.bccancer.bc.ca).
11 Brenner H: Long-term survival rates of cancer patients achieved by the end of the 20th century: a period analysis. Lancet 2002;360:1131–1135.
12 Inskip PD: Multiple primary tumors involving cancer of the brain and central nervous system as the first or subsequent cancer. Cancer 2003;98:562–570.
13 Peterson KM, Shao C, McCarter R, et al: An analysis of SEER data of increasing risk of secondary malignant neoplasms among long-term survivors of childhood brain cancer. Pediatr Blood Cancers 2006; 47:83–88.

Krueger H, McLean D, Williams D: The Prevention of Second Primary Cancers.
Prog Exp Tumor Res. Basel, Karger, 2008, vol 40, pp 32–44

5

Lymphomas

Lymphoma is a general term for a group of cancers that originate in the lymphatic system. There are 2 major categories: Hodgkin's disease [1] and all other types, usually known as non-Hodgkin's lymphoma (NHL). In lymphomas, malignant lymphocytes accumulate due to over-production and/or failure to die, creating a characteristic impact on lymph nodes. The many subgroups of the disease are classified by the exact cell types affected; immunologic and genetic features are also used to specify the different lymphomas [2]. Despite the range of types, key symptoms are shared among the lymphomas, such as painless swelling of lymph nodes, fever and fatigue. Prognosis varies across this class of cancers. The 5-year survival rate for Hodgkin's disease is 85%, while the average for the various NHLs is 58%.

About 9 of 10 lymphoma cases involve NHL. While relatively rare, the intense interest in Hodgkin's disease is driven by 2 factors: it occurs relatively frequently in children and it has a high cure rate. This means there is a cohort of long-term survivors of Hodgkin's disease at risk of developing a SPC. We will cover the issues specific to children later in the monograph and the issues related to adult-onset Hodgkin's disease in the next section of this chapter. But we will start by examining SPCs related to NHL.

Although the lymphomas are rarely studied together in the context of SPC, there is a small pool of literature that does combine Hodgkin's disease and NHL, sometimes also weaving in the story related to blood cell malignancies such as the leukemias. These papers usually refer explicitly to lymphatic and hematopoietic cancers, or to the general category of hematologic cancers. In one study [3], the very precise term 'hematolymphoproliferative malignancy' [4] was employed. The data in that report, however, were distinguished across the main lymphomas and leukemias, so they will be presented in the appropriate sections below.

Non-Hodgkin's Lymphoma

The etiology of the various lymphomas is still under investigation. The known risk factors for NHL, namely, immunosuppression (via HIV infection, transplantation as well as congenital and autoimmune conditions) and pesticide and herbicide exposure, account for only a small proportion of the cases [5]. Infections with agents other than HIV have been implicated in some of the more than 20 subtypes of NHL, but once again these account for only a small percentage of the overall incidence [6]. For reasons that are not entirely clear, rates of NHL have been rising in developed countries in recent years, which places it in the same company as melanoma, but distinct from virtually every other type of cancer [7]. NHL is now the fifth most common malignancy in the world [8].

Ten years ago, the usual treatment for NHL was cytotoxic chemotherapy alone. Today, autologous stem cell transplantation combined with high-dose chemotherapy are routine for aggressive disease. Also, the use of monoclonal antibodies is becoming well established [9]. Finally, radiotherapy has been shown to be effective, at least in early-stage NHL [10].

The most comprehensive research on SPC related to NHL is that conducted by Brennan and colleagues [11]. They examined over 109,000 patients in 13 cancer registries [12]. Based on their study, there was an overall 47% increase (SIR = 1.47; 95% CI 1.43–1.51) in the risk of SPC after NHL, which is reasonably consistent with previous reports [13]. A significantly increased risk was confirmed for cancers that were also noted in earlier research, that is, lung, bladder, kidney, acute nonlymphocytic leukemia [14], Hodgkin's disease and melanoma. Many other sites were also implicated (though more weakly), including lip, tongue, oropharynx, stomach, small intestine, colon, liver, nasal cavity, soft tissues, skin (nonmelanoma), thyroid gland and blood (specifically, acute lymphocytic leukemia). A 'therapy effect' was noted for lung and bladder cancer and acute nonlymphocytic leukemia, as well as for Hodgkin's disease and stomach cancer [15].

Table 10, adapted from Brennan and colleagues, outlines the increased risk of a SPC after NHL. Following the pattern described in chapter 4 (pp 25–31), we ranked the SPCs according to estimated population impact. The SIR by length of follow-up is also provided. These data sometimes demonstrate an increasing risk over time, which is one pattern that researchers identify with a so-called therapy effect. The only SPCs with significant SIRs not included in this table (due to low population impact) are those of the lip, salivary gland, small intestine, nose/nasal cavity, bone, testis and eye.

There has been only modest enhancement of the epidemiologic literature related to NHL and SPC since the 2005 study by Brennan and colleagues. In 2006, Moser and colleagues [18] reported on 748 patients treated for aggressive NHL. Half the patients required salvage treatment, that is, additional chemotherapy and radiotherapy that may increase the risk of SPC. Most died of the primary malignancy before SPC could occur; those with longer survival could develop another cancer and even die from it. Thus, at 15 years of follow-up, the cumulative mortality rate was 11% for solid cancers and 3% for acute myeloid leukemia. Given the effect of the length of survival, it is not surprising that younger patients with aggressive NHL are at the highest risk for SPC. Table 11 summarizes the significant SIRs among patients in the cohort who were under 45 years of age.

Table 10. SPC following NHL by follow-up period

SPC	Overall SIR	Years of follow-up: SIR			
		<1 year	1–4 years	5–9 years	≥10 years
Lung	1.48 (1.38–1.58)	1.26	1.30	1.72	1.78*
Colorectal					
Colon	1.29 (1.18–1.41)	0.97	1.26	1.39	1.51
Brain/Central nervous system	1.35 (1.06–1.69)	1.29	1.02	1.75	1.59
Leukemia					
ANLL	1.52 (1.13–2.00)	1.45	1.60	1.93	0.94
ALL	2.65 (2.21–3.14)	1.99	2.71	3.11	2.59
Other [16]	3.31 (2.64–4.11)	3.54	3.27	3.28	3.24
Esophagus	1.41 (1.13–1.75)	0.80	1.42	1.47	1.98
Stomach	1.34 (1.19–1.50)	1.21	1.27	1.13	1.91*
Kidney	1.94 (1.70–2.21)	5.13	1.08	1.54	1.21
Oral					
Oropharynx	2.22 (1.42–3.30)	3.12	1.86	2.35	1.97
Tongue	2.69 (1.94–3.62)	2.38	3.12	1.61	3.41
Bladder	1.50 (1.35–1.67)	1.24	1.21	1.61	2.21*
Melanoma, skin	1.92 (1.69–2.16)	2.09	2.15	1.86	1.38*
Thyroid gland	2.26 (1.71–2.94)	2.95	1.64	2.07	3.13
Hodgkin's disease	5.14 (4.00–6.50)	3.93	3.54	6.87	7.69*
Liver [17]	1.55 (1.20–1.96)	2.15	1.24	1.29	1.89
Nonmelanoma, skin	3.28 (3.07–3.49)	2.27	3.56	3.99	2.82
Soft tissue sarcoma	2.44 (1.81–3.23)	1.92	1.77	3.20	3.40
All cancers	**1.47 (1.43–1.51)**	**1.36**	**1.37**	**1.55**	**1.67***

Figures in parentheses are 95% CI. ANLL = Acute non-lymphocytic leukemia; ALL = acute lymphocytic leukemia. *Significant trend over time. Adapted from Brennan et al. [11].

Some attention has been paid to specific subtypes within the class of NHLs, including those that occur extranodally (that is, in the skin, stomach, brain, etc.). For example, a small study indicated that patients with nongastric mucosa-associated lymphoid tissue lymphoma are not at increased risk of SPC [19].

A 2007 analysis of 9 population-based US registries extended our understanding of SPC following 2 related variants of a cutaneous T cell lymphoma, namely mycosis fungoides and Sézary syndrome [20]. Cutaneous lymphomas are rare malignancies;

Table 11. SPC following NHL in patients younger than 45 years

SPC	Overall SIR
Lung	15.4 (4.2–39.4)
Colorectal	12.5 (2.6–36.5)
Leukemia	16.7 (1.4–93.1)
Hodgkin's disease	60.1 (12.4–175.3)

Figures in parentheses are 95% CI. Adapted from Moser et al. [18].

Table 12. SPC following mycosis fungoides or Sézary syndrome

SPC	Overall SIR
NHL	5.08 (3.34–7.38)
Melanoma, skin	2.60 (1.25–4.79)
Urinary system	1.74 (1.08–2.66)
Hodgkin's disease	17.14 (6.25–37.26)
All cancers	**1.32 (1.15–1.52)**

Figures in parentheses are 95% CI. From Huang et al. [24].

as a class, they represent about 2% of all lymphomas, with a global incidence of 0.3–1.0 per 100,000 [21]. Mycosis fungoides is the most common cutaneous T cell lymphoma, and in fact accounts for 50% of all primary cutaneous lymphoma [22]. It also seems to be on the increase, which may explain the intensified research focus [23]. Eight of the SEER datasets in the 2007 analysis generated significant SIRs for 4 types of SPC following mycosis fungoides/Sézary syndrome (table 12).

Data from the Stanford registry included in this report confirmed that Hodgkin's disease had the highest excess risk and also suggested that cancers of the biliary system could be added to the list (SIR = 11.76, 95% CI 1.51–42.02) [20]. The notably elevated risk for Hodgkin's disease was confirmed in a 2007 German study based on a small patient series [24]. We also note that the increased risk for melanoma is consistent with earlier reports [25, 26]. Finally, a patient series in Israel suggested that various types of NHL predominate even more than Hodgkin's disease following occurrences of mycosis fungoides [27].

For completeness, we should mention the potential overlap of etiology of at least some cases of mycosis fungoides/Sézary syndrome and adult T cell leukemia/lymphoma, that is, infection with human T cell leukemia virus type 1. However, the role of this virus in mycosis fungoides/Sézary syndrome is still under investigation [28, 29].

Having understood some of the better established SPC associations, it is natural to raise the question of prevention. Interventions addressing the excess risk of SPC generally target one of the proposed causal pathways related in some way to the primary

Table 13. SPC following Non-Hodgkin's Lymphoma NHL (no radiation vs. radiation)

SPC	Overall SIR	No radiation	Radiation
Breast	0.85 (0.78–0.93)	0.79 (0.71–0.88)	1.00 (0.86–1.16)
Mesothelioma [32]	1.22 (0.72–1.93)	0.86 (0.39–1.63)	2.26 (1.03–4.28)
Soft tissue sarcoma	1.78 (1.31–2.36)	1.42 (0.94–2.07)	2.65 (1.62–4.10)
All cancers	**1.14 (1.11–1.17)**	**1.13 (1.10–1.17)**	**1.18 (1.12–1.23)**

Figures in parentheses are 95% CI. Adapted from Tward et al. [30].

cancer. Therapy effects are of particular interest to clinicians, because of the potential for adjusting the intervention and thus lowering the risk of SPC.

Tward et al. [30] studied 77,876 patients who were treated for NHL between 1973 and 2001. A key aspect of their research was to assess the effect of external beam radiation therapy on the development of second malignancies. When all second cancers were considered together, the risk associated with irradiation did not significantly exceed that seen in the unirradiated cohort. The story for specific second primaries was different, however. Irradiated patients showed an excess risk for soft tissue sarcomas and mesothelioma compared with unirradiated survivors. We should note that these are rare cancers, though mesothelioma continues to receive attention in the literature [31]. Finally, Tward and colleagues demonstrated that the risk of second female breast cancer was also significantly higher in irradiated patients; in fact, in unirradiated cases, the cancer rate was actually lower than in the general population (SIR = 0.79). Table 13 provides selected information from the study by Tward and coauthors.

Another point may be raised about second breast cancer in this context, specifically in terms of prognosis. When compared against all second breast cancers, research has revealed that the cases of SPC of the breast following NHL (and following Hodgkin's disease) demonstrate worse outcomes [33].

We could also note that different studies draw disparate conclusions about SPC etiology. Thus, the increase in stomach cancer and (possibly) lung cancer seen earlier in the research by Brennan and colleagues may be due to irradiation, as suggested by rising SIRs over the follow-up period. However, the results of Tward and colleagues did not implicate external beam radiation therapy in either of these SPCs.

Not shown table 13, but included in the full results of the study by Tward and coauthors, was an analysis that looked at the age of primary cancer onset. Patients who were treated prior to the age of 25 years were at higher risk of a SPC than those treated after 25. In the under 25 group, the risk of SPC for those who were irradiated (SIR = 4.51) was higher than for those who were not (SIR = 2.1).

The bi-directionality of some cancer risks (for example, Hodgkin's disease increasing after NHL and vice versa) suggests a common environmental or host factor risk.

With the lymphomas, this seems to relate to a compromised immune system and/or viral infection (for example with Epstein-Barr virus) [11]. For instance, the most likely common denominator of NHL as well as skin, oropharyngeal and liver cancers has been identified as immunosuppression, in some cases exploited by a viral infection [34, 35]. With respect to liver cancer associations, it is of interest that both hepatitis B and C have been linked to the development of certain NHL subtypes [36, 37].

The role of UV radiation in NHL remains under investigation [38, 39]. A positive association seems plausible enough, given that UV light is a potent immunosuppressant, causing damage to DNA in skin cells. However, a recent pooled analysis of 10 case-control studies supported the conclusion that intermittent (that is, recreational, not occupational) sun exposure may actually be protective against NHL, possibly mediated by optimized vitamin D production [40].

Another instance of immunosuppression involves the conditioning regimens used with transplantation to treat NHL (as well as Hodgkin's disease). There are 2 varieties of such treatment, bone marrow grafts and peripheral stem cell transplantation; both are sometimes referred to as hematopoietic stem cell transplantation [41]. The problem is not the graft per se (which is actually quite effective), but rather the chemotherapy before and after, and the associated risk of inducing acute myeloid leukemia. The adjuvant total body irradiation sometimes used in transplantation procedures has also been implicated in the development of SPC [42].

On another iatrogenic front, bladder cancer has been associated with chemotherapy using cyclophosphamide. A smaller study from 2006 further examined the impact of chemotherapy following NHL [43]. An elevated risk for leukemia and possibly lung and colorectal cancer was seen in treated patients, though the relationship between chemotherapy and lung cancer has been questioned in other reports [44]. Generally, the SIRs in this study were greater in patients who were younger at first treatment.

Smoking offers another obvious linkage, especially between NHL, lung cancer and bladder cancer, but in fact it has only been conclusively (though weakly) associated with particular subtypes of NHL [45, 46]. Likewise, alcohol may not be the usual suspect drawn in to explain an association with oropharyngeal cancers, as some studies have actually supported a protective effect for alcohol (especially wine) consumption on the development of NHL [47, 48].

To sum up, based on the best current evidence, the potentially most fruitful preventive measures for SPC following NHL include:

(1) reducing suppression of the immune system (for example, through safer chemotherapy protocols)

(2) not becoming exposed to or infected with new viral triggers.

As different suspect viruses can be present in the host prior to chemotherapy, prevention of SPC may prove difficult in the short run. The development and use of prophylactic vaccines against viruses may be helpful in reducing the rate and impact of such carrier states.

Hodgkin's Disease (Adult Onset)

As the following series of tables demonstrate, Hodgkin's disease in adults continues to be an area of great interest to SPC investigators. The rationale is similar to that driving pediatric Hodgkin's disease research (see chapter 14, pp 122–134), namely, a high cure rate, generating a substantial population of long-term survivors with the potential for SPC development. Mortality associated with Hodgkin's disease has been dramatically reduced since the 1970s. Future progress on survival must take into account the late effects of Hodgkin's disease; this will include targeted prevention of SPC.

Our first evidence concerning appropriate prevention targets comes from a large study (n = 32,591) conducted by Dores and coauthors [49]. The number of SPCs of significant excess risk is remarkable. The 'stand-out' second primaries, calibrated by SIR and position in table 14, are lung cancer, leukemia and NHL. Breast, esophagus, stomach and oropharynx are also notable.

This analysis was updated in 2007 by members of the same research group [51]. They identified 18,862 five-year survivors of Hodgkin's disease from 13 population-based cancer registries in North America and Europe. The conclusions confirmed the excess risk for breast cancer following Hodgkin's disease (SIR = 6.1) and for solid tumors both above (SIR = 6.0) and below (SIR = 3.7) the diaphragm. The largest increase in risk was for malignant mesothelioma, a relatively uncommon cancer. The cumulative risk for SPC at 30 years of follow-up is about 3 times higher in patients with Hodgkin's disease than in the general population. Of concern in terms of secondary prevention, younger Hodgkin's disease patients demonstrated an elevated risk of breast and colorectal cancer prior to the age when routine screening is normally recommended.

As is often true, there are both modifiable and nonmodifiable forces behind SPC development in patients with Hodgkin's disease. The latter category typically includes genetic make-up. In the case of Hodgkin's disease, indirect evidence of a genetic influence on SPC has been gathered through studies of family members; when there is a family history of cancer, the rate of SPC following Hodgkin's disease is higher [52, 53]. More direct evidence of the effect of patient chromosomal instability and certain polymorphisms on SPC rates has also been generated recently [54, 55]. The impact of known genetic factors is generally felt in terms of susceptibility to late effects due to therapy. In fact, the story of SPC prevention in Hodgkin's disease is largely related to therapy, as we will see in the balance of this section.

There are multiple approaches to treating Hodgkin's disease, and most of them demonstrate a certain level of risk related to SPC development. With radiotherapy, complexity in any predictions about 'late effects' partly arises because there are numerous body areas (called fields) that may receive radiation. When directed at the neck, central chest and lymph nodes under the arms, the therapy is referred to as radiation to the mantle field. If radiation is also given to the central lymph nodes in the upper abdomen, the spleen and the pelvis, it is called total nodal irradiation.

Table 14. SPC following Hodgkin's disease

SPC	Overall SIR		
	all patients	males	females
Lung	2.9 (2.6–3.2)	2.7	3.4
Colon	1.6 (1.4–1.9)	1.6	1.7
Breast	2.0 (1.8–2.3)		2.0
Pancreas	1.5 (1.1–2.0)		
NHL	5.5 (4.7–6.4)	5.5	5.6
Brain	1.5 (1.1–2.1)	1.8	
Leukemia	9.9 (8.7–11.2)	9.7	10.2
Acute lymphoblastic leukemia	7.1 (3.6–12.8)	7.9	5.7
Acute myeloid leukemia [50]	21.5 (18.3–25.0)	23.1	18.9
Esophagus	2.8 (1.8–4.0)	2.1	4.7
Stomach	1.9 (1.5–2.4)	2.0	1.8
Kidney	1.5 (1.1–2.1)	1.6	
Oral	2.5 (1.5–4.0)	2.1	3.6
Pharynx	3.3 (2.2–4.9)	3.1	4.1
Urinary bladder	1.4 (1.1–1.8)		1.9
Melanoma, skin	1.7 (1.3–2.3)	2.2	
Cervix	2.0 (1.4–2.7)		2.0
Thyroid gland	4.1 (3.0–5.5)	3.1	4.6
Liver and intrahepatic bile duct	1.6 (1.1–2.3)	1.9	
Connective tissue	5.1 (3.5–7.2)	5.1	5.0
Tongue	2.8 (1.5–4.7)	3.3	
Salivary gland	6.1 (3.5–9.9)	5.0	7.7
Bone	3.8 (1.7–7.2)		7.1
Lip	3.9 (2.4–5.9)	3.3	9.5
All cancers	**2.3 (2.2–2.4)**	**2.2**	**2.3**

Figures in parentheses are 95% CI. Adapted from Dores et al. [49].

When restricted to the femoral, inguinal and pelvic area, the label applied is inverted Y radiotherapy. Another important distinction is whether the radiation is focused on tissues with manifest clinical involvement ('involved-field radiotherapy') or if it encompasses uninvolved areas contiguous with the involved field ('extended-field radiotherapy'). Mantle radiotherapy and other traditional types just described generally fall into the extended-field category. Finally, radiation therapy may be adjuvant to chemotherapy, or vice versa. The various combinations and doses of the 2 types of therapies create many variables to be considered in a full assessment of SPC risk.

Several important findings from the study by Dores and colleagues begin to clarify the situation with respect to therapy and SPC risk. It is not a minor topic of concern. Despite the reputation of Hodgkin's disease being a childhood illness, adult patients with this condition actually 'sustain the greatest second cancer burden' [49]. Based on trends across follow-up periods (not shown in our summary table, see chapter 15, pp 135–137), several cancers seem to be a late effect of radiotherapy. These are the malignancies where the excess risk begins to appear 10 years following Hodgkin's disease diagnosis, and then increase thereafter. The cancers are esophageal, gastric, colorectal, bladder and female breast.

This increase in breast cancer is consistent with many reports of elevated risk of breast cancer after radiation [56]. A recent case-control study confirmed that breast cancer risk increases with the dose of radiation for Hodgkin's disease [57]. The one Cochrane review that focuses on SPC does in fact deal with Hodgkin's disease as the first primary cancer, specially focusing on the effect of treatment [58]. The analyses of 10 randomized controlled trials suggest that the risk of a second breast cancer is over 3 times higher in extended-field radiotherapy compared with involved-field radiotherapy.

Whether other cancers should be on the 'watch list' with respect to radiotherapy remains a matter of investigation. Some researchers have identified lung, thyroid gland and bone as sites also at risk for radiation-induced cancers. Studies have specifically linked lung cancer following Hodgkin's disease to an effect of radiotherapy (and/or chemotherapy) [59, 60]. Data derived by Gilbert et al. [61] in a case-control study in 2003 confirmed that radiation (and/or chemotherapy) for Hodgkin's disease does induce lung cancer, with a radiation dose-response relationship and a multiplication effect when smoking was also involved.

Given the effectiveness of present chemotherapy protocols, radiotherapy has taken somewhat of a backseat in Hodgkin's disease; some have positioned radiation as mainly the strategy for unresponsive or highly localized disease. On the other hand, chemotherapy itself has been linked to increased risk of second lung cancer, as we have just noted, though some reports suggest this relationship only applies when smoking also is a factor [44]. Combining chemotherapy and radiotherapy introduces new complexities. The Cochrane review noted earlier demonstrated that adding radiotherapy to chemotherapy marginally increases SPC risk in advanced stages of primary Hodgkin's disease, compared to initial chemotherapy alone. Adding chemotherapy to initial radiotherapy produced more surprising results. The odds ratio of developing a SPC compared to radiotherapy alone was 0.78 (95% CI 0.62–0.98). The authors explained the protective effect in terms of the lower relapse rate and/or reduced need for more salvage therapy that results from that particular treatment protocol; the hypothesis is that more intensive therapy leads to more SPC, so that avoiding such follow-up leads to fewer second primaries [62]. Interestingly, this positive profile for certain applications of initial radiotherapy runs counter to some of the therapeutic trends in the arena of Hodgkin's disease, and may require a reassessment [63].

As well as the treatments already noted, bone marrow and blood transplantation is sometimes used (especially in recurrent disease). There are also cutting edge approaches under serious investigation, including immunotherapies. The therapeutic options for Hodgkin's disease clearly represent a complex story. An important ongoing theme in that story is the primary prevention of SPC, especially the continued quest for therapies and protocols with a favorable risk/effectiveness profile. As well as introducing novel strategies that may be safer, there are ongoing efforts in the realm of radiotherapy and chemotherapy. This has included moving from extended- to involved-field radiotherapy, adjusting radiation dosage as well as innovations such as intensity-modulated and image-guided radiotherapy [64, 65]. For example, a small 2007 study demonstrated that shifting from extended- to involved-field radiotherapy for Hodgkin's disease reduced second breast and lung cancers in women by 65%; lowering radiation dosage reduced SPC risk even further [66].

To sum up, in the case of many solid SPCs, the main prevention strategy is mostly related to therapy adjustment to avoid serious late effects. The only exception in this story is well known, namely, encouragement to quit smoking to prevent second lung cancer. In other words, the prevention options are limited. Early detection of SPCs seems to be a vital building block in the care for Hodgkin's disease survivors. Researchers have confirmed that significant elevated risks may require a surveillance program for 25 years or more after Hodgkin's disease diagnosis, complemented by 'programs of patient and public awareness' [67]. The long latency period for the most severe late effects poses a challenge both for health care protocols and resources and for epidemiological research to identify SPC risk factors.

The greatest immediate potential for reducing SPC following Hodgkin's disease may have already been introduced, namely, the use of new, safer chemotherapy regimens, typically without adjuvant radiation [68, 69]. The combined modality popular since the 1960s, involving earlier chemotherapy agents and radiation, while offering a high cure rate, has been strongly linked to the occurrence of acute leukemia, a complication that is very often fatal [70]. The newer chemotherapies are very effective when used as a single modality, and to date have resulted in essentially no leukemia development. However, we have seen that the story concerning radiotherapy is not over, with the recent analysis of multiple randomized controlled trials suggesting that modern combination treatments involving initial radiation may be protective against some SPCs. The quest for therapeutic strategies of high effectiveness and safety continues, but clinical education regarding practice recommendations may prove to be even more important [71]. Once safer protocols of reasonable efficacy have been determined, it will be important to facilitate their widespread adoption by clinicians.

Notes and References

1 Named after Thomas Hodgkin, who described cases in 1832. Sometimes an apostrophe is not used for Hodgkin's disease (or non-Hodgkin's lymphoma), that is, the term employed would be Hodgkin disease. Recently, there has been a move to reclassify and relabel Hodgkin's disease as Hodgkin's lymphoma.
2 Harris NL, Jaffe ES, Diebold J, et al: The World Health Organization classification of neoplastic diseases of the hemoatopoietic and lymphoid tissues. Ann Oncol 1999;10:1419–1432.
3 Dong C, Hemminki K: Second primary neoplasms among 53,159 haematolymphoproliferative malignancy patients in Sweden, 1958–1996: a search for common mechanisms. Br J Cancer 2001;85:997–1005.
4 Note also the use of lymphohematopoietic and hematolymphopoietic as aggregate categories in the literature.
5 Vineis P: Incidence and time trends for lymphomas, leukemias and myelomas: hypothesis generation. Working Group on the Epidemiology of Hematolymphopoietic Malignancies in Italy. Leuk Res 1996;20: 285–290.
6 Grulich AE, Vajdic CM: The epidemiology of non-Hodgkin lymphoma. Pathology 2005;37:409–419.
7 Bray I, Brennan P, Boffetta P: Recent trends and future projections of lymphoid neoplasms – a Bayesian age-period-cohort analysis. Cancer Causes Control 2001;12:813–820.
8 Chiu BC, Weisenburger DD: An update of the epidemiology of non-Hodgkin's lymphoma. Clin Lymphoma 2003;4:161–168.
9 Hennessy BT, Hanrahan EO, Daly PA: Non-Hodgkin lymphoma: an update. Lancet Oncol 2004;5: 341–353.
10 Gustavsson A, Osterman B, Cavallin-Stahl E: A systematic overview of radiation therapy effects in non-Hodgkin's lymphoma. Acta Oncol 2003;42:605–619.
11 Brennan P, Scelo G, Hemminki K, et al: Second primary cancers among 109,000 cases of non-Hodgkin's lymphoma. Br J Cancer 2005;93:159–166.
12 US SEER cancer registries were not included, since a separate analysis related to them was already in process.
13 Boffetta P, Butler J, Maynadie M, et al: Lymphomas; in Neugut AI, Meadows AT, Robinson E (eds): Multiple Primary Cancers. Philadelphia, Lippincott Williams & Wilkins, 1999.
14 Also called acute myeloid leukemia or acute myelogenous leukemia.
15 Epidemiological data indicate a 'therapy effect,' sometimes called a 'treatment effect', when there is an increase in risk with increased time since diagnosis of the first primary, and when there is a greater risk at younger age of primary cancer onset (when treatments are likely to be more intensive).
16 Leukemias other than acute lymphocytic leukemia or acute non-lymphocytic leukemia.
17 Although the incidence and proportion of PYLL of liver cancer is relatively low across the population, we include it here because of the mortality implications faced by individual patients. One estimate of 5-year survival with lung cancer was less than 8%, as indicated in table 8.
18 Moser EC, Noordijk EM, van Leeuwen FE, et al: Risk of second cancer after treatment of aggressive non-Hodgkin's lymphoma; an EORTC cohort study. Haematologica 2006;91:1481–1488.
19 Arcaini L, Burcheri S, Rossi A, et al: Risk of second cancer in nongastric marginal zone B-cell lymphomas of mucosa-associated lymphoid tissue: a population-based study from northern Italy. Clin Cancer Res 2007;13:182–186.
20 Huang KP, Weinstock MA, Clarke CA, et al: Second lymphomas and other malignant neoplasms in patients with mycosis fungoides and Sezary syndrome: evidence from population-based and clinical cohorts. Arch Dermatol 2007;143:45–50.
21 Prince HM, McCormack C, Ryan G, et al: Management of the primary cutaneous lymphomas. Australas J Dermatol 2003;44:227–240; quiz 241–242.
22 Keehn CA, Belongie IP, Shistik G, et al: The diagnosis, staging, and treatment options for mycosis fungoides. Cancer Control 2007;14:102–111.
23 Criscione VD, Weinstock MA: Incidence of cutaneous T-cell lymphoma in the United States, 1973–2002. Arch Dermatol 2007;143:854–859.
24 Hallermann C, Kaune KM, Tiemann M, et al: High frequency of primary cutaneous lymphomas associated with lymphoproliferative disorders of different lineage. Ann Hematol 2007;86:509–515.
25 Evans AV, Scarisbrick JJ, Child FJ, et al: Cutaneous malignant melanoma in association with mycosis fungoides. J Am Acad Dermatol 2004;50:701–705.
26 Pielop JA, Brownell I, Duvic M: Mycosis fungoides associated with malignant melanoma and dysplastic nevus syndrome. Int J Dermatol 2003;42:116–122.

27 Barzilai A, Trau H, David M, et al: Mycosis fungoides associated with B-cell malignancies. Br J Dermatol 2006;155:379–386.

28 Shohat M, Shohat B, Mimouni D, et al: Human T-cell lymphotropic virus type 1 provirus and phylogenetic analysis in patients with mycosis fungoides and their family relatives. Br J Dermatol 2006;155: 372–378.

29 Walsh PT, Benoit BM, Wysocka M, et al: A role for regulatory T cells in cutaneous T-cell lymphoma; induction of a CD4+CD25+Foxp3+ T-cell phenotype associated with HTLV-1 infection. J Invest Dermatol 2006;126:690–692.

30 Tward JD, Wendland MM, Shrieve DC, et al: The risk of secondary malignancies over 30 years after the treatment of non-Hodgkin lymphoma. Cancer 2006;107:108–115.

31 Teta MJ, Lau E, Sceurman BK, et al: Therapeutic radiation for lymphoma: risk of malignant mesothelioma. Cancer 2007;109:1432–1438.

32 A tumor affecting the lining of the chest or abdomen.

33 Sanna G, Lorizzo K, Rotmensz N, et al: Breast cancer in Hodgkin's disease and non-Hodgkin's lymphoma survivors. Ann Oncol 2007;18:288–292.

34 Hemminki K, Jiang Y, Steineck G: Skin cancer and non-Hodgkin's lymphoma as second malignancies. markers of impaired immune function? Eur J Cancer 2003;39:223–229.

35 Negri E, Little D, Boiocchi M, et al: B-cell non-Hodgkin's lymphoma and hepatitis C virus infection: a systematic review. Int J Cancer 2004;111:1–8.

36 Wang SS, Cozen W, Cerhan JR, et al: Immune mechanisms in non-Hodgkin lymphoma: joint effects of the TNF G308A and IL10 T3575A polymorphisms with non-Hodgkin lymphoma risk factors. Cancer Res 2007;67:5042–5054.

37 Nieters A, Kallinowski B, Brennan P, et al: Hepatitis C and risk of lymphoma: results of the European multicenter case-control study EPILYMPH. Gastroenterology 2006;131:1879–1886.

38 Smedby KE, Hjalgrim H, Melbye M, et al: Ultraviolet radiation exposure and risk of malignant lymphomas. J Natl Cancer Inst 2005;97:199–209.

39 Armstrong BK, Kricker A: Sun exposure and non-Hodgkin lymphoma. Cancer Epidemiol Biomarkers Prev 2007;16:396–400.

40 Kricker A, Armstrong BK, Hughes AM, et al: Personal sun exposure and risk of non Hodgkin lymphoma: a pooled analysis from the Interlymph Consortium. Int J Cancer 2008;122:144–154.

41 Transplantation may be allogenic, involving tissue from another person, or autologous. Autologous stem cell transplants refer to stem cells that are collected from an individual and given back to that same individual. Autologous transplants are also referred to as autografts or autotransplants. Peripheral blood stem cell transplantation is a new technique in which stem cells are obtained from a patient's blood and used in bone marrow transplantation. Before the transplant is done, the patient receives high-dose chemotherapy and/or radiation therapy to destroy diseased cells. It is this aspect of the overall treatment protocol that may increase SPC risk.

42 Metayer C, Curtis RE, Vose J, et al: Myelodysplastic syndrome and acute myeloid leukemia after autotransplantation for lymphoma: a multicenter case-control study. Blood 2003;101:2015–2023.

43 Mudie NY, Serdlow AJ, Higgins CD, et al: Risk of second malignancy after non-Hodgkin's lymphoma: a British cohort study. J Clin Oncol 2006;24:1568–1574.

44 Amadori D, Ronconi S: Secondary lung tumors in hematological patients. Semin Respir Crit Care Med 2005;26:520–526.

45 Stagnaro E, Tumino R, Parodi S, et al: Non-Hodgkin's lymphoma and type of tobacco smoke. Cancer Epidemiol Biomarkers Prev 2004;13:431–437.

46 Schollkopf C, Smedby KE, Hjalgrim H, et al: Cigarette smoking and risk of non-Hodgkin's lymphoma – a population-based case-control study. Cancer Epidemiol Biomarkers Prev 2005;14:1791–1796.

47 Besson H, Brennan P, Becker N, et al: Tobacco smoking, alcohol drinking and Hodgkin's lymphoma: a European multi-centre case-control study (EPILYMPH). Br J Cancer 2006;95:378–384.

48 Briggs NC, Levine RS, Bobo LD, et al: Wine drinking and risk of non-Hodgkin's lymphoma among men in the United States: a population-based case-control study. Am J Epidemiol 2002;156:454–462.

49 Dores GM, Metayer C, Curtis RE, et al: Second malignant neoplasms among long-term survivors of Hodgkin's disease: a population-based evaluation over 25 years. J Clin Oncol 2002;20:3484–3494.

50 For our purposes, this may be equated with acute non-lymphocytic leukemia.

51 Hodgson DC, Gilbert ES, Dores GM, et al: Long-term solid cancer risk among 5-year survivors of Hodgkin's lymphoma. J Clin Oncol 2007;25:1489–1497.

52 Lorenzo Bermejo J, Sundquist J, Hemminki K: Effect of parental history of cancer on the development of second neoplasms after lymphoma at the same site than the parents. Leukemia 2007, E-pub ahead of print.

53 Landgren O, Pfeiffer RM, Stewart L, et al: Risk of second malignant neoplasms among lymphoma patients with a family history of cancer. Int J Cancer 2007;120:1099–1102.

54 M'kacher R, Bennaceur-Griscelli A, Girinsky T, et al: Telomere shortening and associated chromosomal instability in peripheral blood lymphocytes of patients with Hodgkin's lymphoma prior to any treatment are predictive of second cancers. Int J Radiat Oncol Biol Phys 2007;68:465–471.
55 Worrillow L, Smith A, Scott K, et al: Polymorphic MLH1 and risk of cancer after methylating chemotherapy for Hodgkin lymphoma. J Med Genet 2007, E-pub ahead of print.
56 Boice JD Jr: Radiation and breast carcinogenesis. Med Pediatr Oncol 2001;36:508–513.
57 Van Leeuwen FE, Klokman WJ, Stovall M, et al: Roles of radiation dose, chemotherapy, and hormonal factors in breast cancer following Hodgkin's disease. J Natl Cancer Inst 2003;95:971–980. See also Hill DA, Gilbert E, Dores GM, et al: Breast cancer risk following radiotherapy for Hodgkin lymphoma: modification by other risk factors. Blood 2005;106:3358–3365.
58 Franklin JG, Paus MD, Pluetschow A, et al: Chemotherapy, radiotherapy and combined modality for Hodgkin's disease, with emphasis on second cancer risk. Cochrane Database Syst Rev 2007, issue 4, CD003187. Also see the summary in Franklin J, Pluetschow A, Paus M, et al: Second malignancy risk associated with treatment of Hodgkin's lymphoma: meta-analysis of the randomised trials. Ann Oncol 2006;17:1749–1760.
59 Travis LB, Gospodarowicz M, Curtis RE, et al: Lung cancer following chemotherapy and radiotherapy for Hodgkin's disease. J Natl Cancer Inst 2002;94: 182–192.
60 Swerdlow AJ, Schoemaker MJ, Allerton R, et al: Lung cancer after Hodgkin's disease: a nested case-control study of the relation to treatment. J Clin Oncol 2001;19:1610–1618.
61 Gilbert ES, Stovall M, Gospodarowicz M, et al: Lung cancer after treatment for Hodgkin's disease: focus on radiation effects. Radiat Res 2003;159:161–173. See also van Leeuwen FE, Klokman WJ, Stovall M, et al: Roles of radiotherapy and smoking in lung cancer following Hodgkin's disease. J Natl Cancer Inst 1995;87:1530–1537.
62 Franklin J, Pluetschow A, Paus M, et al: Second malignancy risk associated with treatment of Hodgkin's lymphoma: meta-analysis of the randomised trials. Ann Oncol 2006;17:1749–1760.
63 Yahalom J: Transformation in the use of radiation therapy of Hodgkin lymphoma: new concepts and indications lead to modern field design and are assisted by PET imaging and intensity modulated radiation therapy (IMRT). Eur J Haematol Suppl 2005;66:90–97.
64 Girinsky T, Ghalibafian M: Radiotherapy of hodgkin lymphoma: indications, new fields, and techniques. Semin Radiat Oncol 2007;17:206–222. Although we should note that some of the imaging techniques used in planning and guiding therapy themselves appear to elevate the risk of SPC. See also Beyan C, Kaptan K, Ifran A, et al: The effect of radiologic imaging studies on the risk of secondary malignancy development in patients with Hodgkin lymphoma. Clin Lymphoma Myeloma 2007;7:467–469.
65 Hodgson DC, Koh ES, Tran TH, et al: Individualized estimates of second cancer risks after contemporary radiation therapy for Hodgkin lymphoma. Cancer 2007;110:2576–2586.
66 Koh ES, Tran TH, Heydarian M, et al: A comparison of mantle versus involved-field radiotherapy for Hodgkin's lymphoma: reduction in normal tissue dose and second cancer risk. Radiat Oncol 2007; 2:13.
67 Travis LB, Hill DA, Dores GM, et al: Breast cancer following radiotherapy and chemotherapy among young women with Hodgkin disease. J Am Med Assoc 2003;290:465–475.
68 Friedman DL, Constine LS: Late effects of treatment for Hodgkin lymphoma. J Natl Compr Cancer Netw 2006;4:249–257.
69 Schonfeld SJ, Gilbert ES, Dores GM, et al: Acute myeloid leukemia following Hodgkin lymphoma: a population-based study of 35,511 patients. J Natl Cancer Inst 2006;98:215–218.
70 Longo DL: Radiation therapy in the treatment of Hodgkin's disease – do you see what I see? J Natl Cancer Inst 2003;95:928–929.
71 Gobbi PG, Broglia C, Levis A, et al: MOPPEBV-CAD chemotherapy with limited and conditioned radiotherapy in advanced Hodgkin's lymphoma: 10-year results, late toxicity, and second tumors. Clin Cancer Res 2006;12:529–535.

Krueger H, McLean D, Williams D: The Prevention of Second Primary Cancers.
Prog Exp Tumor Res. Basel, Karger, 2008, vol 40, pp 45–50

6

Leukemias

Leukemia is a form of cancer that begins in the blood-forming cells of the bone marrow. Leukemia, which literally means white blood in Greek, is a condition where there is a chronic excess of abnormal white blood cells in the patient's bloodstream. There are more than a dozen varieties of leukemia, but the following 4 types are the most common:

- acute lymphocytic leukemia [1]
- acute nonlymphocytic leukemia [2]
- chronic lymphocytic leukemia
- chronic myeloid leukemia [3].

Leukemia is often thought to be a childhood disease. In fact, leukemia strikes 10 times as many adults as children. The average age of individuals with chronic lymphocytic leukemia is roughly 70 years, and in chronic myeloid leukemia it is 40–50 years. Acute myeloid leukemia is the most common adult form of leukemia [4]. In contrast, acute lymphocytic leukemia is in fact largely a pediatric disease (see chapter 14, pp 122–134).

Two other blood and bone marrow diseases are important in this context. First, myelodysplastic syndrome refers to a varied group of hematopoietic disorders [5]. The stem cell injury that initiates myelodysplastic syndrome can result from chemotherapy, radiation exposure, viral infection, chemical exposure or genetic predisposition. Of most importance from the perspective of SPC, myelodysplastic syndrome may occur following treatment for certain hematologic cancers [6]. The disease often progresses and can evolve into leukemia.

The second allied condition is multiple myeloma, a relatively rare cancer. It is characterized by the accumulation of malignant plasma cells in the bone marrow and excess immunoglobulin in the serum and/or urine. The disease consists of 4 different molecular subtypes, which may require different therapeutic strategies [7]. The global incidence rate of multiple myeloma is about 3.3 per 100,000 [8].

Depending upon the type of leukemia, there are 5 major treatment approaches:

(1) chemotherapy
(2) interferon therapy to slow the production of leukemia cells and enhance the immune system

Table 15. SPC following lymphoid leukemia by follow-up period

SPC	Overall SIR	Years of follow-up: SIR		
		<1 year	1–9 years	>9 years
Myeloid leukemia	2.46 (1.22–4.42)		3.13	
NHL	3.85 (2.92–4.98)		4.33	3.94
Hodgkin's disease	4.29 (1.83–8.50)		4.60	
Nervous system	1.93 (1.21–2.92)	6.09		3.10
Squamous cell carcinoma, skin	5.28 (4.38–6.31)		6.14	4.33
All cancers	**1.25 (1.16–1.35)**		**1.30**	

Figures in parentheses are 95% CI. Adapted from Dong and Hemminki [11].

(3) radiation
(4) stem cell transplantation, to restore the immune system following treatment with high doses of chemotherapy and radiation therapy
(5) surgery to remove an enlarged spleen
(6) blocking a specific receptor (for example, Gleevec® for chronic myeloid leukemia).

As we saw with lymphomas in the previous chapter, most of these interventions may be a risk factor for SPC. For instance, in bone marrow transplantation, which is used to treat leukemia more than any other condition, the same late effects occur as described in the previous chapter for the lymphomas, namely, an excess of hematologic cancers following the conditioning regimens [9]. This phenomenon suggests the need to use the safest protocols possible and to maintain life-long surveillance during patient follow-up. It is important to note that the risks of SPC related to transplantation appear to be higher in younger patients [10].

Dong and Hemminki [11] combined the primary lymphocytic (or lymphoid) leukemias in a 2001 study of SPCs. They confirmed that SPC risk was largely limited to the hematologic malignancies (table 15). Note that the excess risk of SPC was particularly high for skin cancer and subsequent lymphomas.

Large epidemiologic studies have confirmed that the specific category of chronic lymphocytic leukemia (by definition a longer-term disease) demonstrates increased risk of developing SPC. For example, an analysis of US SEER data suggested that there may be an excess SPC risk related to several solid tumors, including lung, larynx, melanoma and Kaposi sacrcoma [12]. The elevated risk for second lung cancer was also noted in a 2005 study [13]. The most recent analysis evaluated all Danish patients with chronic lymphocytic leukemia from 1943 to 2003 (n = 12,373), with results shown in table 16 [14].

Table 16. SPC following chronic lymphocytic leukemia

SPC	Overall SIR
Lung	1.61 (1.37–1.90)
Breast	0.70 (0.50–0.97)
NHL	2.73 (1.99–3.75)
Kidney	1.84 (1.31–2.58)
Oral/pharynx	1.77 (1.18–2.67)
Melanoma	2.42 (1.66–3.53)
Thyroid	2.64 (1.10–6.35)
Hodgkin's disease	4.95 (2.36–10.4)
Salivary gland	3.36 (1.26–8.95)
Bone	4.26 (1.07–17.0)
Nonmelanoma skin cancer	3.66 (3.32–4.04)
All cancers	**1.59 (1.50–1.69)**

Figures in parentheses are 95% CI. Adapted from Scholkopf et al. [14].

Many of the disease associations remain unexplained. An increased risk was observed for cancer sites where smoking is known to play a role, but researchers have questioned whether it is in any way explanatory [15]. One of the cautions about such an etiologic link is that 'there is little evidence for an association between smoking and [chronic lymphocytic leukemia]' [14].

The impact of chemotherapy for chronic lymphocytic leukemia remains controversial. Some studies have suggested that the late effects following chronic lymphocytic leukemia are independent of the initial treatment used, except perhaps the excess leukemias following certain chemotherapies [16]. Other proposals for the mechanism of increased risk include a common viral or other etiology, overlapping genetic factors and simply the immunodeficiency related to leukemia [17–19].

In the absence of clear SPC etiologies and prevention strategies, close surveillance is advisable during the usually prolonged survival following chronic lymphocytic leukemia. Such surveillance would include a regular skin examination for melanoma and nonmelanoma skin cancers.

Understanding the excess in skin cancer after lymphoid leukemia has been a special focus of research [20]. While UV radiation is clearly an etiologic factor, as the cancers occur in areas of the body where there is maximal sun exposure, the most important driver of excess cases is likely the primary or treatment-related immunodeficiency. Similarly, immunocompromised transplant patients of all types experience more skin cancers (in previously sun-damaged skin) compared with the general population. This reinforces the concept that an intact immune system is of basic importance

Table 17. SPC following hairy cell leukemia

SPC	Overall SIR
Lung	0.63
NHL	5.03
Thyroid	3.56
Hodgkin's disease	6.61
All cancers	**1.24**

Adapted from Hisada et al. [21].

Table 18. SPC following multiple myeloma by follow-up period

SPC	Overall SIR	Years of follow-up: SIR		
		<1 year	1–9 years	>9 years
Myeloid leukemia	8.19 (5.70–11.4)		9.50	7.43
NHL	1.74 (1.12–2.57)		1.78	
Solid tumors	0.81 (0.73–0.90)		0.77	0.73
All cancers	**0.94 (0.86–1.03)**			

Figures in parentheses are 95% CI. Adapted from Dong and Hemminki [11].

in the control of cancer development. It is important to note that there is no evidence for SPC arising through a direct effect on skin DNA by any factor other than past UV exposure [11].

As in NHL, researchers are becoming more focused on leukemia subtypes in order to specify and stratify SPC risks. In 2007, over 3,000 patients with so-called hairy cell leukemia (a rare form of chronic lymphocytic leukemia) were evaluated. A few categories of SPC demonstrated significant SIRs, including all cancers (table 17) [23]. Smaller studies on the SPC impact of specific therapies for leukemia have also recently been pursued [22, 23].

In the study introduced above, Dong and Hemminki also looked at SPC following multiple myeloma. As is often the case with hematologic malignancies, it is hematologic SPC that dominates the story of subsequent cancers (table 18) [24].

Paralleling the situation that has been observed with myeloid leukemia, there actually appear to be fewer solid tumors than expected in the general population. Another report originating in the Nordic region of the world confirmed no excess of solid tumors after chemotherapy for multiple myeloma [25]. In contrast, a study based on

Table 19. SPC following multiple myeloma

SPC	Overall SIR
Colon	1.25 (1.06–1.47)
NHL	1.51 (1.14–2.01)
Bladder	1.42 (1.13–1.78)
Kaposi sarcoma	5.42 (2.51–11.69)

Figures in parentheses are 95% CI. Adapted from Cannon et al. [26].

US SEER data suggested that multiple myeloma patients did demonstrate an excess of second solid tumors at certain sites (table 19) [26].

The most dramatic result was found for Kaposi sarcoma, which is often associated with immunosuppressed transplantation and HIV/AIDS patients. A similar (though nonsignificant) excess risk of Kaposi sarcoma was observed in another study from the same era [27]. The probable explanation for this phenomenon is that Kaposi sarcoma is a sequela of primary or secondary immunosuppression in the presence of pre-existing human herpesvirus-8 infection. This virus is strongly associated with Kaposi sarcoma development in other clinical situations [28].

Notes and References

1 The qualifier lymphoid or lymphoblastic is also used.
2 An alternate term for this disease is acute myeloid leukemia.
3 The qualifier myelogenous is also used.
4 See the information from the American Cancer Society summarized at www.oncologychannel.com/leukemias/index.shtml.
5 Bennett JM, Komrokji RS: The myelodysplastic syndromes: diagnosis, molecular biology and risk assessment. Hematology 2005;10(suppl 1):258–269.
6 Ogasawara T, Yasuyama M, Kawauchi K: Therapy-related myelodysplastic syndrome with monosomy 5 after successful treatment of acute myeloid leukemia (M2). Am J Hematol 2005;79:136–141.
7 Durie BG: The epidemiology of multiple myeloma. Semin Hematol 2001;38(suppl 3):1–5.
8 Phekoo KJ, Schey SA, Richards MA, et al: A population study to define the incidence and survival of multiple myeloma in a National Health Service Region in UK. Br J Haematol 2004;127:299–304.
9 Curtis RE, Travis LB, Rowlings PA, et al: Risk of lymphoproliferative disorders after bone marrow transplantation: a multi-institutional study. Blood 1999;94:2208–2216.
10 Curtis RE, Rowlings PA, Deeg HJ, et al: Solid cancers after bone marrow transplantation. N Engl J Med 1997;336:897–904.
11 Dong C, Hemminki K: Second primary neoplasms among 53,159 haematolymphoproliferative malignancy patients in Sweden, 1958–1996: a search for common mechanisms. Br J Cancer 2001;85:997–1005.
12 Hisada M, Biggar RJ, Greene MH, et al: Solid tumors after chronic lymphocytic leukemia. Blood 2001;98:1979–1981.
13 Amadori D, Ronconi S: Secondary lung tumors in hematological patients. Semin Respir Crit Care Med 2005;26:520–526.
14 Schollkopf C, Rosendahl D, Rostgaard K, et al: Risk of second cancer after chronic lymphocytic leukemia. Int J Cancer 2007;121:151–156.

15 Kyasa MJ, Hazlett L, Parrish RS, et al: Veterans with chronic lymphocytic leukemia/small lymphocytic lymphoma (CLL/SLL) have a markedly increased rate of second malignancy, which is the most common cause of death. Leuk Lymphoma 2004;45:507–513.
16 Morrison VA, Rai KR, Peterson BL, et al: Therapy-related myeloid leukemias are observed in patients with chronic lymphocytic leukemia after treatment with fludarabine and chlorambucil: results of an intergroup study, cancer and leukemia group B 9011. J Clin Oncol 2002;20:3878–3884.
17 Molica S: Second neoplasms in chronic lymphocytic leukemia: incidence and pathogenesis with emphasis on the role of different therapies. Leuk Lymphoma 2005;46:49–54.
18 Landgren O, Pfeiffer RM, Stewart L, et al: Risk of second malignant neoplasms among lymphoma patients with a family history of cancer. Int J Cancer 2007;120:1099–1102.
19 Wiernik PH: Second neoplasms in patients with chronic lymphocytic leukemia. Curr Treat Options Oncol 2004;5:215–223.
20 Levi F, Randimbison L, Te VC, et al: Non-Hodgkin's lymphomas, chronic lymphocytic leukaemias and skin cancers. Br J Cancer 1996;74:1847–1850.
21 Hisada M, Chen BE, Jaffe ES, et al: Second cancer incidence and cause-specific mortality among 3,104 patients with hairy cell leukemia: a population-based study. J Natl Cancer Inst 2007;99:215–222.
22 Tavernier E, Le QH, de Botton S, et al: Secondary or concomitant neoplasms among adults diagnosed with acute lymphoblastic leukemia and treated according to the LALA-87 and LALA-94 trials. Cancer 2007;110:2747–2755.
23 Au WY, Kumana CR, Lam CW, et al: Solid tumors subsequent to arsenic trioxide treatment for acute promyelocytic leukemia. Leuk Res 2007;31:105–108.
24 For more on this topic, see the overview in Leone G, Mele L, Pulsoni A, et al: The incidence of secondary leukemias. Haematologica 1999;84:937–945.
25 Wang CC, Chen ML, Hsu KH, et al: Second malignant tumors in patients with nasopharyngeal carcinoma and their association with Epstein-Barr virus. Int J Cancer 2000;87:228–231.
26 Cannon MJ, Flanders WD, Pellett PE: Occurrence of primary cancers in association with multiple myeloma and Kaposi's sarcoma in the United States, 1973–1995. Int J Cancer 2000;85:453–456.
27 Iscovich J, Boffetta P, Winkelmann R, et al: Classic Kaposi's sarcoma as a second primary neoplasm. Int J Cancer 1999;80:178–182.
28 Tedeschi R, Kvarnung M, Knekt P, et al: A prospective seroepidemiological study of human herpesvirus-8 infection and the risk of multiple myeloma. Br J Cancer 2001;84:122–125.

Krueger H, McLean D, Williams D: The Prevention of Second Primary Cancers.
Prog Exp Tumor Res. Basel, Karger, 2008, vol 40, pp 51–55

7

Breast Cancer (Female)

Breast cancer is the most common cancer in women of developed countries. A large percentage of women diagnosed with breast cancer survive for an extended period of time. They are at risk of developing a new primary cancer, which has implications both for long-term follow-up and for research into common etiologies.

We note from the start that an important decision in any epidemiologic investigation of breast cancer is whether or not a new contralateral breast tumor will be included in SPC statistics.

Taking advantage of the growing number of cancer registries, many large studies of SPC risk following breast cancer have been published. A literature review of this work was conducted in 2006 by Mellemkjaer et al. [1], revealing the following pattern:

- an overall SIR of 1.20–1.30 (not including contralateral breast cancer)
- the most consistent reports were found for excess cancer of the endometrium, ovary, thyroid gland and lung as well as soft tissue sarcomas and leukemia
- there is some evidence of higher risk of melanoma and cancers of the stomach and colon following female breast cancer.

Mellemkjaer and colleagues augmented the past research with their own analysis of 525,527 primary breast cancer cases drawn from 13 population-based cancer registries outside the US. The overall SIR was 1.25 (95% CI 1.24–1.26), consistent with previous studies. The risk was positively correlated with time since breast cancer diagnosis, but decreased with higher age at diagnosis of the first primary.

The results for specific second primary sites are shown in table 20 (including significant data from different follow-up periods, in some cases indicating trends). Although Mellemkjaer and colleagues chose not to focus on second breast cancer, the highest risk for subsequent cancer is in fact related to new primary tumors in the same or contralateral breast. A recent study showed a SIR as high as 3.5 for such malignancies following a first primary breast cancer [3].

By comparison, Raymond and Hogue [4] presented results from the US SEER database. They found a significantly elevated risk of both second breast and non-breast cancer that continued for at least 20 years after the initial breast cancer. In their study, the risk for both types of plural cancer increased with a younger age at diagnosis

Table 20. SPC following breast cancer by follow-up period

SPC	Overall SIR [2]	Years of follow-up: SIR		
		<1 year	1–9 years	≥10 years
Lung	1.24		1.08	1.68
Colorectal	1.22		1.22	1.30
NHL				1.39
Ovary	1.48	1.32	1.38	1.75
Leukemia				
ANLL	1.52		2.28	2.11
Esophagus			1.27	2.09
Stomach	1.35		1.34	1.49
Kidney	1.27			
Oropharynx			1.16	1.40
Urinary bladder			1.16	1.30
Melanoma, skin	1.29			
Uterus	1.52			
Thyroid gland	1.62			
Nonmelanoma skin	1.58	1.23	1.55	1.77
Soft tissue sarcoma				
Thorax/upper limb	2.25		4.73	10.75
All cancers	**1.25**	**1.04**	**1.20**	**1.42**

ANLL = Acute nonlymphocytic leukemia. Adapted from Mellemkjaer et al. [1].

of the first primary. Women who had their initial breast cancer between the ages of 20–29, for example, had a SIR of 48.4 for a second breast cancer and 8.90 for a second non-breast cancer at 10 years of follow-up.

A slightly larger study by Brown et al. [5] was published in 2007, with data drawn from 4 Nordic cancer registries also used by Mellemkjaer and coauthors. The main differences in the new analysis are that the authors omitted hematologic cancers and that the follow-up period was extended to 30 years. The significant overall results are shown in table 21.

Not surprisingly, there is good overlap in the data from the 2 studies using multiple (sometimes overlapping) registries, especially over the first dozen or so SPCs. A new

Table 21. SPC following breast cancer

SPC	Overall SIR
Lung	1.25
Colon	1.12
Rectum/anus	1.13
Pancreas	1.07
Ovary	1.38
Esophagus	1.44
Stomach	1.28
Kidney	1.13
Urinary bladder	1.07
Melanoma, skin	1.21
Cervix	0.91
Uterus	1.41
Thyroid	1.48
Liver	0.79
Connective tissue	1.80
Small intestine	1.20
Pleura	1.42
Gallbladder	0.88
Brain and nervous system	1.07
Salivary gland	1.35
Bone	1.91
Nonhematologic cancers	**1.15**

Adapted from Brown et al. [5].

feature in the report by Brown and colleagues was an apparent protective effect for cervical, liver and gallbladder cancer, a result that was not discussed in the paper. The other recent research in this area has been very focused on the topic of second breast cancers [6–8].

From the point of view of prevention, it is important to understand the etiologic themes in the SPC risk profile following female breast cancer. The data from the large study by Mellemkjaer and coauthors underlined a likely role for breast cancer treatment in the development of SPC at certain sites. Thus, radiotherapy seems to be implicated in leukemia, in cancers of the esophagus, stomach and lung, and especially in soft tissue sarcomas of the thorax and upper limbs (including the shoulder) – in other words, in sites close to the breast and thus subject to a substantial radiation dose. These associations are supported by multiple studies [9–13]. Thyroid cancer, though considered to be radiation induced, did not demonstrate the expected latency pattern or therapy effect that would support such an etiology.

The study by Mellemkjaer and colleagues confirmed one of the most serious posited consequences of breast cancer chemotherapy, namely, the excess occurrence of acute nonlymphocytic leukemia. By comparison, recent research into the effects of family breast cancer history suggested that acute lymphocytic leukemia (and endometrial cancer) following breast cancer may in fact have a heritable cause [14].

Hormone therapy, often used to treat estrogen receptor-positive breast cancer, has been implicated in excess second endometrial cancers [15, 16]. The study by Mellemkjaer and colleagues did not completely support this idea, instead pointing to the potential importance of common risk factors, whether genetic, reproductive or obesity related. One piece of circumstantial evidence for their assertion is that an increased risk of breast cancer was also seen following endometrial cancer. This bi-directional pattern of risk elevation is also seen with ovarian cancer, which can share certain disease susceptibilities with breast cancer related to germline mutations in genes BRCA1 and BRCA2. While Brown and colleagues expressed more confidence about a role for tamoxifen-based hormone therapy in elevated rates of uterine cancer, their data in this regard were actually as equivocal as those seen in the study by Mellemkjaer and coauthors.

In sum, the most beneficial preventive measure against SPC after primary breast cancer focuses on management of radiotherapy approaches, including ongoing technological advances to limit toxicity by minimizing radiation exposure. The new protocols include improved techniques for whole-breast irradiation (for example, hypofractionation and intensity-modulated radiation therapy) and for irradiating a smaller portion of the breast in a shorter period of time (for example, accelerated partial breast irradiation) [17]. It is not yet clear how the new approaches to radiation may affect late effects such as excess SPC outside the breast.

In the midst of so many unknowns, it is comforting to find a (familiar) prevention message: smoking cessation is recommended to avoid smoking-related cancers subsequent to breast cancer [18]. Indeed, different studies have suggested that the carcinogenic effect of radiotherapy for breast cancer is multiplied in smokers and perhaps even codependent on smoking [19].

When cancer susceptibility genes are present, thorough genetic counseling is now highly recommended, possibly via referral to a hereditary cancer program in a major cancer treatment center. If warranted by the risk assessment, there should be a discussion of risk reduction procedures, including bilateral mastectomy to prevent a second breast cancer, or the prophylactic removal of ovaries to prevent the ovarian cancer that has been associated with the pertinent genes. At the least, such patients could be offered an aggressive surveillance program. The appropriate management ultimately depends on effective genetic testing and adequate counseling resources [20].

Notes and References

1 Munich Mellemkjaer L, Friis S, Olsen JH, et al: Risk of second cancer among women with breast cancer. Int J Cancer 2006;118:2285–2292.

2 The 95% CI for included data (presented graphically in the paper by Mellemkjaer and colleagues) indicated that the included results presented here were in fact significant.

3 Soerjomataram I, Louwman WJ, Lemmens VE, et al: Risks of second primary breast and urogenital cancer following female breast cancer in the south of the Netherlands, 1972–2001. Eur J Cancer 2005;41: 2331–2337.

4 Raymond JS, Hogue CJ: Multiple primary tumours in women following breast cancer, 1973–2000. Br J Cancer 2006;94:1745–1750.

5 Brown LM, Chen BE, Pfeiffer RM, et al: Risk of second non-hematological malignancies among 376,825 breast cancer survivors. Breast Cancer Res Treat 2007;106:439–451.

6 Cardis E, Hall J, Tavtigian SV: Identification of women with an increased risk of developing radiation-induced breast cancer. Breast Cancer Res 2007; 9:106.

7 Trentham-Dietz A, Newcomb PA, Nichols HB, et al: Breast cancer risk factors and second primary malignancies among women with breast cancer. Breast Cancer Res Treat 2007;105:195–207.

8 Decensi A, Zanardi S, Argusti A, et al: Fenretinide and risk reduction of second breast cancer. Nat Clin Pract Oncol 2007;4:64–65.

9 Roychoudhuri R, Evans H, Robinson D, et al: Radiation-induced malignancies following radiotherapy for breast cancer. Br J Cancer 2004;91: 868–872.

10 Yap J, Chuba PJ, Thomas R, et al: Sarcoma as a second malignancy after treatment for breast cancer. Int J Radiat Oncol Biol Phys 2002;52:1231–1237.

11 Kirova YM, Vilcoq JR, Asselain B, et al: Radiation-induced sarcomas after radiotherapy for breast carcinoma: a large-scale single-institution review. Cancer 2005;104:856–863.

12 Rubino C, Shamsaldin A, Le MG, et al: Radiation dose and risk of soft tissue and bone sarcoma after breast cancer treatment. Breast Cancer Res Treat 2005;89:277–288.

13 Kirova YM, Gambotti L, De Rycke Y, et al: Risk of second malignancies after adjuvant radiotherapy for breast cancer: a large-scale, single-institution review. Int J Radiat Oncol Biol Phys 2007;68:359–363.

14 Hemminki K, Zhang H, Sundquist J, et al: Modification of risk for subsequent cancer after female breast cancer by a family history of breast cancer. Breast Cancer Res Treat 2007, E-pub ahead of print.

15 Matesich SM, Shapiro CL: Second cancers after breast cancer treatment. Semin Oncol 2003;30: 740–748.

16 Rubino C, de Vathaire F, Shamsaldin A, et al: Radiation dose, chemotherapy, hormonal treatment and risk of second cancer after breast cancer treatment. Br J Cancer 2003;89:840–846.

17 Keisch M, Vicini F: Applying innovations in surgical and radiation oncology to breast conservation therapy. Breast J 2005;11(suppl 1):S24–S29.

18 Ford MB, Sigurdson AJ, Petrulis ES, et al: Effects of smoking and radiotherapy on lung carcinoma in breast carcinoma survivors. Cancer 2003;98: 1457–1464.

19 Prochazka M, Hall P, Gagliardi G, et al: Ionizing radiation and tobacco use increases the risk of a subsequent lung carcinoma in women with breast cancer: case-only design. J Clin Oncol 2005;23:7467–7474.

20 Ray JA, Loescher LJ, Brewer M: Risk-reduction surgery decisions in high-risk women seen for genetic counseling. J Genet Couns 2005;14:473–484.

Krueger H, McLean D, Williams D: The Prevention of Second Primary Cancers.
Prog Exp Tumor Res. Basel, Karger, 2008, vol 40, pp 56–61

8

Lung Cancer

Apart from 'low-mortality' skin cancers, lung cancer is the most common cancer in the world. Even with improvements in therapy, the 5-year survival rate is still as low as 15% [1]. Among the pool of long-term survivors, there is a risk of late development of a second primary tumor.

There are many framing issues related to the topic of primary lung cancer and SPC. One important question involves whether or not to include new primary lung cancers as part of the discussion of SPC. Multiple primary pulmonary tumors represent a complex topic in their own right, comprising synchronous cases (tumors detected or resected simultaneously) or metachronous occurrences following a primary tumor in the lung or some other site. The latter types need to be classified as either recurrence/metastasis after noncurative therapy or as a true second primary developing independently from the initial cancer. Further criteria relevant to SPC incidence include whether or not the cancer is bilateral, the actual tissue type(s) involved, and the staging of the first primary at the point of detection and therapy [2]. There is great variation in the prognosis related to the various clinical scenarios, one of a number of reasons that this has become a key focus of care in long-term lung cancer survivorship [3].

A further complexity affecting our review is the overlap in the literature between lung malignancies and the broader cancer categories related to the thorax or the upper aerodigestive tract [4]. The latter topic in turn overlaps with another well-studied classification in oncology, namely, head and neck cancers (see chapter 9, pp 62–84). Research has confirmed that, after second lung cancer itself, a primary tumor in the head, neck or upper aerodigestive region of the body is the type of malignancy most often seen in the survivors of primary lung cancer [5, 6].

In this chapter, we focus on cancers following lung cancer proper, as this will be more useful than broader investigative categories such as thoracic cancer. Further, we will be mostly interested in subsequent cancers beyond the lung. Restricting the discussion to non-lung second primaries represents significant scoping, as studies show that over 30% of second primaries following lung cancer are in fact new pulmonary tumors [5, 6]. One advantage of not entering into the topic of second cancer in the

Table 22. SPC following lung cancer

SPC	Overall SIR	
	men	women
Pharynx	1.99 (1.09–3.34)	
Larynx	2.49 (1.87–3.23)	25.17 (8.17–58.70)
Kidney	1.60 (1.23–2.05)	
Urinary bladder	1.94 (1.63–2.28)	
All cancers	**1.07 (1.00–1.14)**	**1.21 (1.02–1.42)**

Figures in parentheses are 95% CI. Adapted from Teppo et al. [7].

lung itself is that we avoid the uncertainty around evaluating how many subsequent cancers in the lung are really new primaries rather than recurrences [7]. It is also important to note that, whatever the cumulative prevalence, the SIR for second lung cancers may be relatively modest. A 1999 study (n = 5,794) suggested that there was a significant excess of second primary pulmonary tumors only in men, with a SIR of 1.6 (95% CI 1.1–2.3) [8].

On the other hand, a focus on non-pulmonary second cancers leaves less to talk about. It seems that the number of sites outside the lung with a statistically significant excess risk of SPC following primary lung cancer is very limited. The 1999 study cited earlier only found an excess of oropharyngeal cancers (SIR 2.7, 95% CI 1.5–4.5) [9]. A 2001 study confirmed this figure, but only in males. In that research, Crocetti et al. [10] also found a SIR of 2.1 (95% CI 1.4–3.0) for cancer of the larynx in male lung cancer survivors.

These results may be compared with the largest sample examined from the same time period, which we adopt as our index results for this chapter of the monograph. Table 22 summarizes the significant data obtained by Teppo et al. [7] from 77,548 lung cancer patients in the Finnish Cancer Registry:

The results demonstrate reasonable consistency with the other reports we have cited. The main exception is that the data for oral cancer were not significant in the Finnish study, though it is possible that the pharynx dominated the oropharyngeal statistics noted in the other papers, thus aligning them better with the study by Teppo and colleagues. This sort of ambiguity can always occur when body sites are combined in different ways in different studies. A new result in the Finnish research was the fact that excess cancers also showed up in the urinary tract. The most dramatic datum, the high SIR for laryngeal cancer in women, is a departure from the conclusions of other studies; no explanation is offered by the authors for a SIR over 25 in this one instance, when the ratio for all second cancers is just over 1. Indeed, it must be acknowledged that the modest SIR reported for all cancers in both men and women barely achieved statistical significance. Finally, we note that the research in this case did not support an excess risk of second primary lung cancer.

How do these data compare with earlier reports? The US SEER figures up to 1994 were analyzed by Ahsan et al. [11] The results suggested a significant excess risk for head and neck cancer (consistent with the study by Teppo and colleagues), as well as esophageal and prostate cancer. Breast cancer occurred in excess only among limited subsets of patients, and specifically not in the cases where lung cancer had been treated by radiation. The reason for the latter, somewhat counterintuitive phenomenon may be that high mortality seen in lung cancer does not accommodate the usual latency period for new cancer development following radiotherapy.

We need to address a final complexity in the epidemiology in this area. Put simply, all primary lung cancers are not the same. The most studied distinction is between small cell and non-small cell lung cancer. According to a review of older research, SPC following small cell lung cancer exhibits the following characteristics: a clear impact of treatment (either radiation or chemotherapy) on SPC rate, highest SPC rates in the aerodigestive tract itself (especially the lung), increasing annual SPC rates and a major reduction in SPC incidence after smoking cessation [12].

The focus on second primaries following non-small cell lung cancer seems to have intensified recently, though the information is still quite limited [13–15]. For instance, we did not locate any research that calculated the excess risks of developing a second cancer. The studies generally have been based on small patient series. The largest one comprised 860 patients [5]. In the latter study, while the proportion of second lung cancers was still high, tumors were also found in a wide range of other sites. The predominant sites in this inventory, that is, head and neck as well as urinary tract epithelium, are closely related to the risk factor of tobacco use.

Recent investigations have included specific types of lung cancer. For instance, 1,182 cases with carcinoid cancer, a type of neuroendocrine tumor, were examined in 2006, revealing a relevant SPC story for both women and men [16]. The risk of second breast cancer was significantly elevated for 5 years after diagnosis, but a protective effect was seen in longer follow-up. On the other hand, prostate cancer occurred 2.8 times more often than expected based on 5 years of follow-up. Genetic predispositions or hormonally related exposures have been posited to explain these effects.

There are 4 dynamics involved with SPC following lung cancer that are crucial to 'positioning' it as a prevention priority. First, the high frequency of primary lung cancer means that even a modest excess risk will translate into a large absolute number of SPC cases. Second, the annual risk of SPC remains constant (or increases) throughout the life of a 'cured' upper aerodigestive tract cancer patient, so vigilance must be maintained throughout follow-up. Third, there is the unfortunate irony that SPC poses the greatest threat in cases of early-stage primary tumors, that is, among patients with the best prognosis for long survival of the first cancer. And, finally, when the second cancer is contracted, it can be quickly fatal. In one study of 1,371 small cell lung cancer patients, the median survival time after contracting a metachronous cancer was only 4 months [17]. The latter dynamic must be assessed in light of the changing balance of histological cancer types in a population [18].

To sum up, the following conclusion, originally derived in reference to upper aerodigestive tract cancers, applies to lung tumors in particular: as early detection, diagnosis and treatment continue to translate into prolonged survival, the lifetime risk of SPC rises concomitantly [12]. This underscores the importance of discovering and applying prevention measures. Although not our main focus, we also note that MPCs in the lung have a high incidence, are diagnosed relatively late and exhibit very poor prognosis. As a consequence, developing effective early detection and treatment strategies for these cancers has also assumed a high priority.

We suggested earlier that the most important categories of non-pulmonary SPC following lung cancer include the head and neck (especially the upper aerodigestive tract); the next most common site is the epithelium of the urinary system. The SIRs summarized in table 22 confirm that these 2 categories represent the cancers with the strongest claim to excess occurrence following a first primary lung tumor. Further, Duchateau and Stokkel [5] have pointed out that the pertinent second primaries are all smoking related. This naturally leads to the possibility of primary prevention of SPC through abstaining from tobacco use [19].

The theoretical foundation for the latter hypothesis has been labeled 'field cancerization'. This is the process whereby the epithelial lining of the upper aerodigestive tract is 'continuously exposed to tobacco and/or alcohol leading to increased risk for multiple independent tumor development that can occur synchronously or metachronously' [12]. Some researchers would object to coordinating alcohol exposure as a concern equivalent to tobacco use; the strongest evidence for alcohol-related risk appears to be limited to esophageal cancer [20]. We also note that a similar field cancerization process may be at work in the case of tobacco-related urinary carcinogens leading to bladder cancer.

Whatever the biological mechanism, a retrospective review of 540 small cell lung cancer patients in 1993 showed that smoking cessation is associated with a significant decrease (over 60%) in risk for a smoking-related SPC [21]. Avoiding tobacco use appears to be the most effective means to prevent SPC following lung cancer, though some studies have shown that risks remain higher in former smokers compared to patients who never smoked [12].

The other potentially modifiable risk factor for SPC following lung cancer is thoracic irradiation (in the context of small cell primary cancer). At this point, it is not clear how much such treatment could be adjusted without affecting survival following the primary cancer. Recent innovations such as three-dimensional conformal and intensity-modulated radiation therapies have unknown implications for SPC development. At the least, 'potential signs and symptoms of thoracic malignancies should be approached with heightened vigilance in any patient who has a history of radiation exposure' [22].

Chemoprevention has been of special interest in upper aerodigestive cancers. Retinoids, natural and synthetic derivatives of vitamin A, produced encouraging results in earlier research. In a 1993 randomized controlled trial, 307 patients with a history of resected stage I non-small cell lung cancer received either 12 months of treatment with retinol palmitate (300,000 IU/day) or no treatment. At a median of 46 months of follow-up, patients in the retinol palmitate arm of the study had a significantly lower incidence of SPC than the control group (3.1 vs. 4.8%) [23]. More recent studies have been less convincing. A study published in 2000 did not reproduce the results noted above, though there was a significant difference in time to development of SPC that favored the retinoid treatment group [24]. Research interest has not abated, but the results continue to be discouraging. A 2001 report of isotretinoin treatment versus control among 1,166 stage I non-small cell lung cancer patients indicated that overall rates of SPC or mortality did not improve, and that the agent was actually harmful in current smokers [25]. A similar harmful effect of β-carotene on smokers has also been demonstrated [26].

We noted already that clinicians know where to look for potential SPC following lung cancer. Progress has been made in detecting early head and neck malignancies, which may also be applied to secondary prevention of SPC in this region of the body. We will further address this important topic, as well as the management of early-stage head and neck cancer, in the next chapter.

Notes and References

1 Brenner H: Long-term survival rates of cancer patients achieved by the end of the 20th century: a period analysis. Lancet 2002;360:1131–1135.

2 Keller SM, Vangel MG, Wagner H, et al: Second primary tumors following adjuvant therapy of resected stages II and IIIa non-small cell lung cancer. Lung Cancer 2003;42:79–86.

3 Sugimura H, Yang P: Long-term survivorship in lung cancer: a review. Chest 2006;129:1088–1097.

4 In particular, the lung is often lumped together with the bronchus in cancer discussions.

5 Duchateau CS, Stokkel MP: Second primary tumors involving non-small cell lung cancer: prevalence and its influence on survival. Chest 2005;127:1152–1158.

6 Liu YY, Chen YM, Yen SH, et al: Multiple primary malignancies involving lung cancer-clinical characteristics and prognosis. Lung Cancer 2002;35:189–194.

7 Teppo L, Salminen E, Pukkala E: Risk of a new primary cancer among patients with lung cancer of different histological types. Eur J Cancer 2001;37:613–619.

8 Levi F, Randimbison L, Te VC, et al: Second primary cancers in patients with lung carcinoma. Cancer 1999;86:186–190.

9 Ibid.

10 Crocetti E, Buiatti E, Falini P: Multiple primary cancer incidence in Italy. Eur J Cancer 2001;37:2449–2456.

11 Ahsan H, Insel BJ, Neugat AI: Risk estimates for second primary cancers; in Neugut AI, Meadows AT, Robinson E (eds): Multiple Primary Cancers. Philadelphia, Lippincott Williams & Wilkins, 1999.

12 Wu X, Hu Y, Lippman SM: Upper aerodigestive tract cancers; in Neugut AI, Meadows AT, Robinson E (eds): Multiple Primary Cancers. Philadelphia, Lippincott Williams & Wilkins, 1999.

13 Kim DJ, Lee JG, Lee CY, et al: Long-term survival following pneumonectomy for non-small cell lung cancer: clinical implications for follow-up care. Chest 2007;132:178–184.

14 Takigawa N, Kiura K, Segawa Y, et al: Second primary cancer in survivors following concurrent chemoradiation for locally advanced non-small-cell lung cancer. Br J Cancer 2006;95:1142–1144.

15 Kawaguchi T, Matsumura A, Iuchi K, et al: Second primary cancers in patients with stage III non-small cell lung cancer successfully treated with chemoradiotherapy. Jpn J Clin Oncol 2006;36:7–11.
16 Cote ML, Wenzlaff AS, Philip PA, et al: Secondary cancers after a lung carcinoid primary: a population-based analysis. Lung Cancer 2006;52:273–279.
17 Soria JC, Brechot JM, Lebeau B, et al: Second primary cancers after small-cell lung cancer. Bull Cancer 1997;84:800–806.
18 Wahbah M, Boroumand N, Castro C, et al: Changing trends in the distribution of the histologic types of lung cancer: a review of 4,439 cases. Ann Diagn Pathol 2007;11:89–96.
19 Rubins J, Unger M, Colice GL: Follow-up and surveillance of the lung cancer patient following curative intent therapy: ACCP evidence-based clinical practice guideline (2nd edition). Chest 2007;132(suppl):355S–367S.
20 Layke JC, Lopez PP: Esophageal cancer: a review and update. Am Fam Physician 2006;73:2187–2194.
21 Richardson GE, Tucker MA, Venzon DJ, et al: Smoking cessation after successful treatment of small-cell lung cancer is associated with fewer smoking-related second primary cancers. Ann Intern Med 1993;119: 383–890.
22 Zablotska LB, Angevine AH, Neugut AI: Therapy-induced thoracic malignancies. Clin Chest Med 2004;25:217–224.
23 Pastorino U, Infante M, Maioli M, et al: Adjuvant treatment of stage I lung cancer with high-dose vitamin A. J Clin Oncol 1993;11:1216–1222.
24 Van Zandwijk N, Dalesio O, Pastorino U, et al: EUROSCAN, a randomized trial of vitamin A and N-acetylcysteine in patients with head and neck cancer or lung cancer. For the European Organization for Research and Treatment of Cancer Head and Neck and Lung Cancer Cooperative Groups. J Natl Cancer Inst 2000;92:977–986.
25 Lippman SM, Lee JJ, Karp DD, et al: Randomized phase III intergroup trial of isotretinoin to prevent second primary tumors in stage I non-small-cell lung cancer. J Natl Cancer Inst 2001;93:605–618.
26 Omenn GS, Goodman GE, Thornquist MD, et al: Risk factors for lung cancer and for intervention effects in CARET, the Beta-Carotene and Retinol Efficacy Trial. J Natl Cancer Inst 1996;88:1550–1559.

Krueger H, McLean D, Williams D: The Prevention of Second Primary Cancers.
Prog Exp Tumor Res. Basel, Karger, 2008, vol 40, pp 62–84

9

Cancers of the Head and Neck

Head and neck cancer is a standard category under which researchers capture information related to both basic science and clinical practice. This aggregation of cancers mainly arose because of common etiology (see below) and the frequency with which cancer in one location spreads to another part of the head or neck. These same factors have made head and neck a catch-all label for an extensive literature on the topic of SPC. This approach creates a challenge for any reviewer, as the information for specific head and neck sites of interest, including the larynx, pharynx and oral cavity, must be abstracted from combined reports and laid alongside other research particular to a site. As a further complexity, some researchers collect information under a heading that is close but not identical to head and neck, namely, the upper aerodigestive tract [1]. Finally, cancers may occur in different tissues in this region of the body. The convention seems to be that, unless otherwise stated, head and neck cancer refers to squamous cell carcinoma of mucosal surfaces.

When the subsequent cancer is itself in the head or neck region, it is not always clear that it is a true second cancer. As we have seen, this 'definitional dilemma' is not unique to the head and neck region. However, researchers of cancer in this part of the body have been at the forefront of the quest to distinguish true SPC from clonal varieties with a common cellular origin [2]. For instance, a molecular means to separate true SPCs has been proposed by Braakhuis and colleagues [3]. The current state of the art posits 3 pathways for the development of second tumors in the head and neck [4]:

(1) Via micrometastases (clonal).
(2) From a common carcinogenic field, yielding so-called second field tumors (partially clonal). We introduced another term for this process earlier, namely, field cancerization, which denotes an epithelial surface marked by 'preneoplastic' genetic alteration. Prolonged exposure of the field to a carcinogen such as tobacco smoke leads to further genetic alteration and ultimately tumor development [5, 6].
(3) Via fully separate clones in different carcinogenic fields (that is, 'true' SPCs that do not originate from the precancerous clone of the first cancer). The latest research suggests that the majority of metachronous cancers fall into this category [7].

Genetic studies will increasingly help to resolve whether synchronous multiple tumors in 1 or more body site are truly independent or have a common clonal origin [8–10]. Such analysis is important because the treatment options related to, for instance, second primary lung cancer are different from those employed in cases involving metastasis of head and neck carcinomas to the lung [11].

Treatment failures in head and neck tumors are often connected to the appearance of second tumors [12]. In developed countries, SPC has been reported in up to 20% of patients with a history of first primaries in the head or neck. However, a large UK study published in 2003 seemingly reported more modest results: multiple cancers in 5.5% of men and 3.6% of women with a first primary. However, applying a Kaplan-Meier analysis that takes into account survival from other causes of death, the SPC rates actually translated into 20% of female cases and 30% of male cases after 20 years [13].

More importantly, the respective SIRs in the UK research were 1.14 (95% CI 1.09–1.19) in males and 1.34 (95% CI 1.24–1.44) in females, allowing the following conclusion: 'a statistically significant higher proportion of subjects diagnosed with a head and neck cancer experienced a new cancer over the study period compared with the general population' [14]. The study further revealed that the AER for cancer [15] subsequent to a first primary was highest in the following sites (in descending order): the pharynx, the oral cavity and the nose/larynx/trachea. This result was largely confirmed by US results published in 2006 (n = 44,862) [16]. Overall, the UK research indicated that second primary sites with significant SIRs following a head or neck cancer were mostly found in the head or neck itself (table 23). Note that, other than the lung, the only exceptions to this rule were found in women and involved stomach as well as bone cancer.

These data may be further compared to the site-based prevalence of SPC following head and neck cancer. A review of 15 studies (n = 22,354) demonstrated that 46% of SPCs were in the head and neck itself, 23% in the lung and 9% in the esophagus [11]. In absolute terms, lung cancer by far accounted for the highest number of excess second cancer cases in head and neck cancer survivors (both male and female). A US SEER study confirmed the excess risk of lung cancer following head and neck cancer [17], as did a smaller series published in 2004 [18]. In sum, 'lung cancer mortality and mortality from other tobacco-associated diseases are major causes of death in people who have survived 1 head and neck cancer' [13].

Reviewers have underlined the urgency of a prevention program, given that development of a second malignancy following head and neck cancer usually has such a poor prognosis [19]. Where to begin such a program? First, it is important to note that if one eliminates the tobacco-associated sites from the large UK study that yielded our index statistics, the SIR for the remaining cancers combined is not significant. This fact yields strong circumstantial evidence that a common environmental cause, namely, tobacco exposure, is the driving force behind excess SPC following head and neck cancers [20]. Thus, smoking cessation is a potentially effective prevention approach, as suggested in a 2007 report [21]. However, the direct evidence related to this hypothesis has been

Table 23. SPC following head and neck cancer

SPC	Overall SIR	
	men	women
Lung	1.45 (1.35–1.56)	2.41 (2.08–2.79)
Esophagus	2.15 (1.79–2.58)	3.53 (2.62–4.74)
Stomach		1.55 (1.14–2.12)
Oral	5.56 (4.11–7.52)	15.31 (10.70–21.89)
Oropharynx	4.67 (3.01–7.24)	8.82 (3.96–19.64)
Tongue	4.20 (2.92–6.04)	5.78 (3.11–10.74)
Larynx		4.52 (2.35–8.69)
Hypopharynx	2.90 (1.68–4.99)	6.25 (2.81–13.91)
Nasopharynx	5.24 (2.82–9.73)	8.57 (2.76–26.58)
Salivary gland	2.82 (1.52–5.25)	5.77 (2.59–12.84)
Thyroid gland		2.87 (1.43–5.73)
Lip		6.90 (1.72–27.58)
Bone		6.15 (2.31–16.40)
All cancers	**1.14 (1.09–1.19)**	**1.34 (1.24–1.44)**

Figures in parentheses are 95% CI. Adapted from Warnakulasuriya et al. [13].

mixed. An earlier study showed no improvement in excess risk with smoking (or drinking) cessation [22]. On the other hand, research published a decade later suggested that former smokers did enjoy a decreased risk of SPC [23]. Finally, a 2003 study agreed with the earlier, more conservative estimates of prevention potential. The authors of the latter report concluded that the impact of smoking history could not easily be reversed, in other words, there already was 'a critical cellular level of cumulative and persistent damage' [24]. While stopping smoking is still important, the evidence of lingering tissue damage leads to the strong conclusion that dissuading people from starting tobacco use in the first place is of paramount importance in cancer control.

Interestingly, a general link between radiotherapy and excess SPC of the head and neck as a whole has not been demonstrated [25, 26]. A recent report confirmed this result across all cancer subsites and also concluded that adding chemotherapy does not influence the incidence of SPC one way or another [27]. A 2005 study added detail to the general picture, demonstrating that there was a low risk of SPC following irradiation of lymphoma in the head and neck [28]. Contrary evidence does exist. Apparently, there is a small risk of developing a variety of radiation-induced soft tissue sarcomas [29]. And, as will be described in a later section, radiotherapy for oral cancer may be a risk factor for SPCs.

There is also evidence of a genetic predisposition for SPC (especially of the oropharynx) among younger survivors of head and neck cancer [30, 31]. While such risk factors are presently not modifiable, this information may eventually be used to guide therapeutic and prevention decisions [32, 33]. At the very least, the focus and intensity of surveillance efforts may produce an increased understanding of the genetic basis for SPC.

Studies on the chemoprevention of SPC related to the head and neck have yielded mixed evidence [34]. Thus, the use of antioxidant agents such as β-carotene remains experimental [13, 35, 36]. Vitamin A and N-acetylcysteine were ineffective in reducing the risk of SPC in one study [37]. Somewhat driven by the lack of alternatives, intensive research continues in the field of chemoprevention, with some promise being shown by combination regimens that target specific molecular defects [38, 39]. It seems, however, that there is a long way to go before success is announced. Concerns about toxicity frequently arise, and efficacy remains elusive. For instance, recent randomized trials have not demonstrated the effectiveness of isotretinoin (13-*cis* retinoic acid) or α-tocopherol in controlling SPC; in fact, the latter agent actually was found to increase second cancer incidence [40–42].

A final etiologic and prevention category has been generating a great deal of interest. Human papillomavirus (HPV) DNA has been detected in a variety of head and neck cancers [43]. Specific sites of interest include the larynx, the tonsils and the oral cavity [44]. Data supporting a link between HPV and oropharyngeal cancers are the most compelling [45]. Pertinent to our topic, Hemminki and colleagues have shown consistent increases in second HPV-related cancers, including oral cancers, when the first cancer was itself HPV-related [46]. The growing evidence suggests a possible role for HPV eradication or vaccination in the control of SPC following a first cancer of the head and neck.

Given the volume of SPC following head and neck cancer, interventions on all high-risk behaviors (mainly related to smoking and drinking) and surveillance of 'at least the adjacent tobacco-associated cancer sites' [13] seem prudent. A UK review in the late 1990s concluded that, on balance, primary prevention may hold out the most hope, at least in the case of oral cancer, since there was 'insufficient evidence to recommend population screening' [47] for that type of malignancy. However, in contrast to universal screening, the targeted surveillance that can be applied after a first primary head and neck cancer may yet prove effective and even cost-effective [48].

In terms of secondary prevention, detection of SPC localized in the head or neck is usually possible through panendoscopy. Because the risk of developing SPC is constant over many years, patients with head and neck cancer essentially 'should be followed up forever' [49]. There continues to be an intense search for reliable biomarkers to detect subclinical disease and allow early intervention for SPC [50, 51].

Upper Aerodigestive Tract

As noted earlier, the term upper aerodigestive tract is also used as an umbrella covering various subsites, many of which overlap with the head and neck. Before turning to

Table 24. SPC following upper aerodigestive tract cancers

SPC	Overall SIR	
	men	women
Upper aerodigestive tract	7.51 (6.60–8.52)	32.93 (26.15–40.94)
Lung	3.14 (2.82–3.49)	4.94 (3.62–6.59)
Colon	1.48 (1.23–1.77)	
Rectum	1.54 (1.23–1.91)	
Pancreas	1.47 (1.09–1.94)	
NHL	1.45 (1.06–1.93)	3.26 (1.99–5.05)
Esophagus	7.02 (5.63–8.65)	9.43 (4.49–17.42)
Stomach	1.38 (1.10–1.71)	
Kidney	1.39 (1.03–1.84)	
Urinary bladder	1.61 (1.35–1.91)	2.09 (1.04–3.75)
Liver	1.96 (1.51–2.51)	
Female genitals [54]		4.00 (1.71–7.92)
Skin	4.59 (4.02–5.21)	6.54 (4.80–8.70)
Nervous system	1.74 (1.22–2.41)	2.14 (1.10–3.74)
Connective tissue	2.53 (1.44–4.11)	
All cancers	**1.92 (1.84–2.01)**	**2.18 (1.97–2.40)**

Figures in parentheses are 95% CI. Adapted from Li and Hemminki [53].

specific subsites of interest, we will briefly review the more modest body of literature related to the upper aerodigestive tract. The sites normally included under this designation are head and neck, lung as well as esophagus [52]. First primary lung cancer was covered in the preceding chapter of this monograph.

Substantive research on SPC following upper aerodigestive tract cancers was published in 2003 by Li and Hemminki [53]. The significant SIRs identified for second tumors are summarized in table 24.

The key linkage between many of these cancers is etiological. Tobacco use is strongly associated with carcinogenesis in both first primaries of the upper aerodigestive tract and in many cases of SPC [55, 56]. Smoking cessation, or not taking up the behavior in the first place, is certainly recommended as a preventive measure. Furthermore, the actual epidemiological impact of smoking cessation after diagnosis remains debatable for many types of SPC following upper aerodigestive tract cancer. A similar ambivalency in the data was already noted for head and neck cancers.

Given the limitations attached to classic primary prevention options, a lot of attention is being paid to chemoprevention to reverse precursor disease or otherwise interrupt carcinogenesis. The key target is high-risk patients, that is, those with a history of upper aerodigestive tract cancer [57]. Such approaches have not yet qualified as standard therapy [58]. Another avenue of investigation has focused on the role of HPV leading to carcinomas in different parts of the aerodigestive tract; the preventive opportunities afforded by vaccination and other measures have become an important part of the discussion [59].

Head and Neck/Upper Aerodigestive Tract Subsites

The anatomy of the head and neck, especially related to the aerodigestive tract, is complex. Many subsites are identified for research purposes, but delineating the borders within what really amounts to a contiguous mucosal surface is problematic. This accounts for the variety of aggregate sites that show up in the literature. While there are studies of index cancers in discrete sites such as the oral cavity, larynx and esophagus, a focus on oropharyngeal malignancy as a first primary is not uncommon. As well, the larynx is often combined with the hypopharynx [60]. The categories can get very elaborate, for example, mouth plus mesohypopharynx. Discussion of the pharynx alone is rare, but research has been conducted in relation to the nasopharynx. Studies also sometimes treat the esophagus and hypopharynx together as a first primary site, or the esophagus and the thyroid gland. Research on SPC following lip or tongue cancer appears to be limited.

In the following brief review of subsites and associated SPCs, we will cover lip and tongue under the first category that deals more or less with the mouth area, that is, the oral cavity proper and the oropharynx. We have elected to include the esophagus in this chapter, even though it can also be classified under the gastrointestinal tract. As well, though it is sometimes handled in its own right as a species of endocrine gland malignancy, there is good reason to include thyroid gland cancer in this part of the monograph. Finally, for convenience, we have incorporated recent data on SPC following ocular melanoma in the last section of this chapter.

Oral Cavity and Oropharynx

Second primary tumors frequently occur following oropharyngeal cancer. Breaking it down further, a smaller study showed that the incidence of SPC ranged from a high of 15% in pharyngeal cancer survivors to a low of 3% among lip cancer patients. The oral floor, oral cavity and tongue fell somewhere in between [61]. A somewhat larger study in Scotland offered the following data concerning significant excess risks of SPC after an index cancer in the oral cavity (table 25) [62].

The dominance of the oral cavity itself as the site of SPC is consistent with other reviews [63]. Earlier research also demonstrated an excess of lip, esophageal and lung cancers following oropharyngeal cancer [64–66]. In addition, studies of cancer registries in the 1980s pointed to an excess risk of tongue cancer [67].

Table 25. SPC following oropharyngeal cancer

SPC	Overall SIR	
	men	women
Oral cavity	108.0 (55.0–185.0)	198.0 (39.5–356.0)
All cancers	**1.95 (1.65–2.24)**	**2.29 (1.70–2.90)**

Figures in parentheses are 95% CI. Adapted from Crosher and McIlroy [62].

Evidence continues to accumulate suggesting that increased fresh fruit or vegetable intake might be effective in preventing oral cancer. Combining this with the fact that the greatest cancer risk following oral cancer is localized in the oral cavity itself, diet offers the potential for some level of SPC control [68, 69]. By comparison, the evidence for chemoprevention is as mixed as that seen for head and neck cancers taken as a whole [70].

On another front, there generally has been little concern about the risks of radiotherapy in head and neck cancers. The one exception may be radiation for oral carcinomas, where elevated risk for head and neck cancers has been observed after a 10-year latency period [71]. Thus, future modifications to treatment protocols may have some impact on SPC development [72].

Overall, it must be admitted that innovation in preventing SPC following oral cancer has been limited. The conclusion of a 1994 report still holds true: 'avoidance of tobacco smoking and alcohol drinking is the most desirable way [...] to reduce the risk of second cancers' [73].

Information on components related to the oropharynx is not extensive. The lip has received some attention. The Scottish report summarized above showed increased risk for nonmelanoma skin cancer and (in men) lip cancer following a first primary cancer of the lip, in other words, in exposed parts of the body. There is good evidence that exposure to sunlight is a risk factor in lip cancer development. This same mechanism may contribute to the elevated SPC rates after lip cancer [74]. Thus, sun protection may represent a preventive avenue. We should note that earlier reports based on the Danish cancer registry also pointed to an elevated risk of oropharyngeal cancer following lip cancer, with the common risk factor of tobacco use being a likely cause [67].

As mentioned earlier, the research on SPC following tongue cancer is especially limited. A 20-year-old study suggested that oropharyngeal cancer risk was 116 times higher in tongue cancer survivors [75]. The prognosis (including SPC development) may be worse for primary tumors at the base of the tongue compared with oral tongue carcinomas, indicating the need for intensified, and targeted, surveillance [76].

Table 26. SPC following cancer of the salivary glands

SPC	Overall SIR
Lung	1.86 (1.45–2.35)
Prostate	1.42 (1.05–1.87)
Head and neck	3.60 (2.31–5.36)
Oral	3.27 (1.19–7.12)
Tongue	3.95 (1.27–9.22)
Salivary gland	7.38 (1.99–18.90)
Thyroid gland	3.31 (1.07–7.73)
All cancers	**1.33 (1.19–1.48)**

Figures in parentheses are 95% CI. Adapted from Sun et al. [78].

Finally, the main result around first primary cancer of the pharynx proper is its strong association with second esophageal cancer, especially the variety that may be characterized as multicentric [65, 77].

Salivary Glands

Limited research has been conducted on SPC following cancer of the salivary glands. A US review based on SEER cases (n = 4,250) yielded the following data concerning excess risks (table 26) [78].

Deviating somewhat from these population-based results, a 2005 retrospective cohort study of 439 female patients with salivary gland tumors indicated that there was a 2.5 times increased risk of second breast cancer. The increased risk for lung cancer shown above was not confirmed in the more recent study, but the dominance of head and neck SPC, and especially oral SPC, was consistent with the earlier report. As well, there was a good match in terms of results for all cancers (SIR = 1.6, 95% CI 1.1–2.3) [79].

Theories concerning cancer associations and the salivary glands involve the 'usual suspects' of tobacco and alcohol consumption as well as dietary factors, though other carcinogens, for example, viruses, are also being investigated. A novel approach attempting to link salivary gland, oral and breast cancers examined the role of Epstein-Barr virus; ultimately, though, the pertinent 2005 study was forced to conclude that there is no 'clear biological explanation for the increased occurrence of second primary breast cancers in patients who have had first primary salivary gland tumours' [80]. Recent work on other viral agencies has been more encouraging. One possibility is connected to Sjögren's syndrome, an uncommon disease involving autoimmunity mechanisms and lymphoproliferation in salivary glands that can lead

Table 27. SPC following nasopharyngeal cancer by follow-up period

SPC	Overall SIR	Years of follow-up: SIR			
		0–2 years	3–5 years	5–10 years	>10 years
Leukemia	9.0 (1.9–26.3) [86]	14.6			
Stomach	5.5 (2.2–11.4)	8.5		9.1	
Head and neck	16.5 (10–26.8)	2.5	19.1	27.7	76.5
All cancers	**2.8 (2–3.9)**	**2.8**	**2.2**	**3.3**	**10.1**

Figures in parentheses are 95% CI. Adapted from Wang et al. [85].

to frank lymphomas. The disorder has generated special interest among cancer researchers and virologists. Most importantly for our purposes, a subset of cases presenting with symptoms similar to Sjögren's syndrome have been connected to both hepatitis C virus infection and B cell lymphomas in different body sites [81].

Nasopharynx

Second primary tumors following nasopharyngeal cancer are rare, and an excess risk has not been observed in some earlier studies [82]. Indeed, in certain patient series, no cases of SPC were detected [27, 48]. A study published in 2000 (see below) did find an increased relative risk of 2.8 for SPC, comparable to the result in an earlier report (SIR = 2.1) [83]. Mechanisms of SPC development have been investigated, including radiotherapy and Epstein-Barr virus infection, but no definite conclusions have been reached [84]. Table 27 provides data from the year 2000 research that indicate a distinctive and even dramatic therapy effect, that is, increasing risk with time after the intervention, at least for SPC of the head and neck [85].

A major population-based update of the information related to nasopharyngeal carcinoma was published in 2007 [87]. Scelo and colleagues examined data from first primary nasopharyngeal carcinoma cases (n = 8,947) in cancer registries from Singapore and 12 other, low-incidence areas. Their work confirmed the associations seen previously (except for second gastric cancer), and expanded the list of SPC demonstrating significant excess risk (table 28).

While this study does represent an improvement in the knowledge base, the authors still recognized certain limitations. Small numbers of specific SPCs may lead to chance associations, and misclassification of recurrences as second cancers, or vice versa, may have over- or underestimated some SIRs. For the most part, the various unproven etiologic hypotheses were not further elucidated. Neither immune suppression nor shared

Table 28. SPC following nasopharyngeal carcinoma

SPC	Overall SIR
Upper aerodigestive tract	3.33 (1.77–5.70)
NHL	3.06 (1.58–5.35)
Tongue	5.29 (1.09–15.5)
Nervous system/brain	3.89 (1.68–7.66)
Nonmelanoma skin cancer	3.47 (2.31–5.02)
Myeloid leukemia	3.85 (1.05–9.86)
All cancers	**1.46 (1.27–1.67)**

Figures in parentheses are 95% CI. Adapted from Scelo et al. [87].

Table 29. SPC following laryngeal cancer

SPC	Overall SIR
Lung	3.56 (3.34–3.79)
Esophagus	3.99 (3.29–4.83)
Head and neck	4.81 (4.31–5.58)
All cancers	**1.68 (1.58–1.79)**

Figures in parentheses are 95% CI. Adapted from Gao et al. [89].

risk factors were confirmed as playing a role, though it is still possible that common genetic mechanisms are involved with second lung tumors and hematologic cancers. Given the strong association of Epstein-Barr virus with nasopharyngeal carcinoma, it was surprising not to find excess risk attached to other Epstein-Barr virus-related cancers, apart from NHL. The best progress on causation maybe came with second tongue cancer. Five of the nine cases occurred 10 years or more after first primary diagnosis, suggesting they may be radiation-induced malignancies. This conclusion was confirmed in an earlier study [88]. Overall, however, very little light has been shed to date on primary prevention targets for SPC following nasopharyngeal carcinoma.

Larynx

Laryngeal carcinoma is a relatively common malignancy in the upper aerodigestive tract, as are subsequent cancers. The largest population-based study used SEER data (n = 20,074). There was an excess risk for all cancers combined, generated especially by tumors localized in the upper aerodigestive tract (table 29) [89].

Table 30. SPC following laryngeal cancer

SPC	Overall SIR
Lung	4.29 (3.2–5.7)
Esophagus	4.43 (1.8–9.1)
Oral or pharynx	7.09 (4.4–10.7)
Thyroid gland	14.02 (2.8–41.0)
All cancers	**1.72 (1.4–2.0)**

Figures in parentheses are 95% CI. Adapted from Levi et al. [100].

The risk factors for developing a SPC following laryngeal carcinoma remain unclear. There was a significant but slight relative risk for radiotherapy across all cancers (1.10) and for lung cancer (1.18). The most convincing therapy risk involved head and neck cancers (1.68, 95% CI 1.16–2.43) in laryngeal cancer survivors. Taking the type of excess SPCs at face value, however, the main etiologic culprit appears once again to be field cancerization synergized by long-term carcinogenic exposure (notably involving tobacco smoke).

Much smaller European registries from the same era (2002–2003) provide useful comparisons for SPC following laryngeal cancer. Analysis in 2 Swiss cantons generated the following data (n = 689; table 30) [90].

This study offered strong support for the SEER results, as well as fine-tuning the differential effect of the specific location of the first primary in the larynx. It seems that cancers occurring outside the glottis proper were a stronger predictor of second primaries. In fact, a 2006 study concluded that the low cumulative incidence of head and neck cancers following glottic cancer did not appear to support routine upper endoscopy [91]. A Slovenian study (n = 2,275 males) offered similar results, with good stratification by follow-up period (table 31) [92].

Note that the conclusion drawn earlier in this chapter for the head and neck region seems to apply to laryngeal cancer, that is, there is no evidence of a therapy effect.

A final prevention issue involves the age at first primary diagnosis. One study concluded that laryngeal cancer patients under 40 years of age experience SIRs for second upper aerodigestive tract cancers that are 2–3 times higher than the figures reported in general populations [93]. Such data, consistent with results developed for first primaries in upper aerodigestive tract as a whole, suggest the need for targeted surveillance in younger laryngeal cancer patients [94].

Esophagus

The relative risk of SPC following cancer of the esophagus has not been a prominent topic in recent research. Most work has focused on the incidence or cumulative

Table 31. SPC following laryngeal cancer by follow-up period

SPC	Overall SIR	Years of follow-up: SIR			
		0–1 year	1–4 years	5–9 years	10–14 years
Lung	4.15 (3.50–4.80)	4.04	4.34	3.90	4.59
Esophagus	4.66 (2.60–7.60)	5.78	5.70	4.64	
Oral cavity	10.07 (6.00–15.70)	29.18	5.32	7.95	8.90
Oropharynx	9.67 (6.20–14.30)	12.51	7.14	9.12	9.96
Tongue	15.97 (9.90–24.10)	30.26	10.90	10.90	18.85
Hypopharynx	6.07 (2.60–11.90)	23.06		8.50	
Lip	5.84 (2.30–12.00)				
All cancers	**2.83 (2.50–3.10)**	**4.36**	**2.68**	**2.40**	**2.59**

Figures in parentheses are 95% CI. Adapted from Ecimovic and Pompe-Kirn [92].

Table 32. SPC following cancer of the esophagus

SPC	Overall SIR	
	men	women
Oral	11.87 (6.62–18.64)	19.61 (6.19–40.56)
Esophagus	10.81 (3.89–21.20)	14.75 (1.39–42.27)

Figures in parentheses are 95% CI. Adapted from Hemminki et al. [46].

incidence of second cancers, which offers no indication about excess risk [95, 96]. The studies dealing with SIRs that we could locate were published just before and just after the key review, *Multiple Primary Cancers,* which summarized research data before 1999. The reason for the limited data may be explained by the following comment found in *Multiple Primary Cancers:* '[second tumors] are virtually unknown because esophageal cancer generally is diagnosed in very advanced stages, and diagnosis is followed very closely by death of the patients' [97].

Table 32 is based on research by Hemminki and colleagues [46]. The connection between esophageal and oral cancers is once again thought to involve the common carcinogenic effects exerted on mucosa by tobacco smoking and alcohol drinking, 2 risk factors that may in fact work synergistically [98, 99].

The most recent update of information concerning esophageal cancer was published by a well-known Swiss research group in 2007 [100]. It was based on first primary cases

Table 33. SPC following esophageal cancer

SPC	Overall SIR
Lung	6.5 (4.3–9.6)
Oral/pharyngeal	57.3 (44.4–72.7)
Larynx	24.3 (11.1–46.2)
Intestine	6.5 (1.2–4.7)
All cancers	**3.7 (3.1–4.3)**

Figures in parentheses are 95% CI. Adapted from Levi et al. [100].

(n = 1,672) drawn from registries in 2 cantons. The significant data are contained in table 33. Previous results were essentially confirmed. The main new result is the extension of (presumably) smoking-related respiratory tract cancer risk to include the lung.

From a secondary prevention point of view, it is most important to detect SPC as early as possible in patients cured of their esophageal cancer. In such patients, it is the subsequent cancer that typically causes death [101, 102]. Thus, follow-up of a first esophageal cancer may need to be intensive and long-term (assuming the initial therapy is successful), incorporating proactive surgical intervention for any subsequent malignancies [103].

The one etiologic factor that has emerged recently is the effect of radiotherapy for the first esophageal cancer. In a 2006 study, the SPC rates were significantly elevated in patients after 15 years, but only in those treated by radiation (SIR = 2.3, 95% CI 1.4–5.4) [104].

Thyroid Gland

Compared to esophageal cancer, the investigation of SPC following thyroid cancer has been extensive. Two very large patient pools were analyzed recently, one US based and one international in scope. A 2005 study of the SEER database offered the following risk assessment in almost 30,000 thyroid cancer patients from over a quarter century (table 34) [105].

The most interesting finding in this study may be that the risk of smoking-related malignancies (notably in the lung) is decreased. This can possibly be attributed to the known low rate of smoking among thyroid cancer patients [106]. It is important to note that both tracheal and scrotal cancers are absolutely rare. The excess salivary gland cancers again may be attributed to radiation effects, but this remains a matter for investigation. The strongest such relationship has been found for leukemia, where there was only a modestly increased SIR. We should note, however, that a therapy effect with respect to leukemia was not borne out by the other recent 'large-sample' investigation, to which we will now turn.

Table 34. SPC following cancer of the thyroid gland

SPC	Overall SIR
Lung	0.87 (0.76–0.99)
Female breast	1.21 (1.11–1.32)
Brain and central nervous system	1.54 (1.09–2.12)
Prostate	1.31 (1.16–1.48)
Leukemia	1.39 (1.07–1.79)
Kidney	2.26 (1.80–2.79)
Salivary gland	2.78 (1.48–4.75)
Scrotum	8.13 (1.63–23.75)
Trachea	14.47 (4.66–33.77)
All cancers	**1.11 (1.06–1.15)**

Figures in parentheses are 95% CI. Adapted from Ronckers et al. [105].

A 2006 survey examined 39,000 thyroid cancer patients across 13 registries from Australian and Canadian provinces, Singapore and several European countries (table 35) [107]. This study did not confirm the SEER result for lung, trachea, brain or scrotum, but did offer a consistent story concerning SPC of the female breast, prostate and salivary glands. There was a stronger indication of excess risk for leukemia following thyroid cancer. Interestingly, the therapy effect suggested here in the case of breast cancer has not been entirely supported by other studies (see below).

The last individual study we will cite in detail was based on a smaller pool (n = approx. 7,000) of thyroid cancer cases. The unique focus of the research in this instance was endocrine malignancies [46]. As table 36 indicates, there was very strong support for the results summarized above for leukemia and cancers of the prostate and brain/central nervous system; good consistency was also evident with respect to the kidney, small intestine and other endocrine glands.

Smaller series with less statistical power have produced more limited results that demonstrate varying levels of agreement with the studies we have already cited. In 2004, Berthe and colleagues analyzed a sample of 875 patients and established a significant SIR of 3.31 for genitourinary tract SPC (in women) [110]. A recent, much larger study of women from the California Cancer Registry confirmed the result for kidney cancer seen above, and also added melanoma as a malignancy with excess risk following thyroid cancer [111].

Radioiodine is the accepted treatment for thyroid cancer. The I-131 isotope circulates throughout the body and is eliminated via the urinary tract, digestive tract and salivary glands, offering many possibilities for potentially carcinogenic exposure. In addition to the role of radiation in leukemia and salivary gland cancer noted earlier, a recent study suggested a dose-response relationship between I-131 ablation and various second cancers, including soft tissue and bone sarcomas as well as colorectal

Table 35. SPC following thyroid cancer by follow-up period

SPC	Overall SIR	Years of follow-up: SIR		
		<1 year	1–9 years	≥10 years
Colorectal	1.27 (1.14–1.42)			
Colon	1.30 (1.13–1.48)			
Rectum	1.23 (1.02–1.47)			
Female breast	1.31 (1.21–1.43)	1.17 (NS)	1.23	1.43
NHL	1.68 (1.37–2.04)	4.78	1.36 (NS)	1.51
Brain and central nervous system	1.39 (1.01–1.87)			
Prostate	1.52 (1.32–1.75)	2.12	1.36	1.59
Leukemia	2.26 (1.85–2.74)	1.99 (NS)	2.36	2.20
Stomach	1.22 (1.01–1.46)			
Kidney	2.33 (1.95–2.76)	6.02	1.75	2.28
Oropharynx	1.43 (1.10–1.84)			
Pharynx	1.72 (1.05–2.66)			
Salivary gland	3.15 (1.76–5.19)			
Endocrine gland [108]	6.75 (3.86–11.0)	19.90	5.01	6.17
Adrenal gland	8.34 (4.16–14.9)	26.90	4.54 (NS)	9.15
Bone	3.62 (1.81–6.48)			
Soft tissue sarcoma	3.63 (2.58–4.96)	4.14	2.95	4.35
Small intestine	2.11 (1.18–3.48)			
Nonmelanoma skin	1.42 (1.19–1.67)	2.34	1.32	1.34
All cancers	**1.31 (1.26–1.36)**	**1.61**	**1.25**	**1.33**

Figures in parentheses are 95% CI. NS = Not significant. Adapted from Sandeep et al. [107].

cancer [112, 113]. By contrast, a 2005 report found only 2 significant risk associations for radiotherapy in thyroid cancer, that is, myeloid leukemia and the upper digestive system [114]. It is not clear what prevention implications flow from this etiologic analysis, apart from the need for targeted surveillance after thyroid cancer treatment. The intensity of such follow-up remains an open question. For instance, the most recent studies that we located actually suggested there was no elevated cancer risk following radioiodine for thyroid carcinoma [115, 116].

Several researchers have focused on female breast cancer as a sequela of thyroid cancer. For example, a 2003 study based on 7,711 thyroid cancer patients found no relationship between radiation dose and SPC of the breast [117]. Another study

Table 36. SPC following thyroid cancer by follow-up period

SPC	Overall SIR	Years of follow-up: SIR		
		<1 year	1–10 years	>10 years
Prostate	1.7 (1.3–2.2)			2.2 (1.5–3.1)
Leukemia	2.3 (1.6–3.2)			2.8 (1.7–4.2)
Kidney	1.9 (1.3–2.6)	12.6 (5.7–22.1)		
Small intestine	3.0 (1.1–5.9)			
Endocrine gland [109]	6.5 (5.2–7.9)	115.4 (87.1–147.6)	3.8 (2.4–5.5)	
Nervous system	1.7 (1.1–2.3)	5.7 (1.5–12.6)		
All cancers	**1.5 (1.4–1.6)**	**6.3 (5.3–7.5)**	**1.3 (1.1–1.4)**	**1.3 (1.1–1.4)**

Figures in parentheses are 95% CI. Adapted from Hemminki and Jiang [46].

focusing on an Israeli population came to the same conclusion [118]. Research based on a smaller sample (n = 2,189) indicated that breast cancer occurred at a significantly elevated risk only in female thyroid cancer patients under 45 years of age [119]. Another intriguing possibility under investigation is the biologic role for thyroid hormone in the etiology of breast carcinoma [120]. While uncertainty about mechanisms linking the 2 cancers continues, most authorities agree that watching for breast cancer is warranted in premenopausal women who have survived thyroid cancer [121, 122].

Confirming the perception of general concern and the specific SPC risk across a variety of sites, in 2007, Subramanian and colleagues conducted a systematic review and meta-analysis of the published literature related to thyroid cancer [123]. They pooled data from 2 studies we have already summarized plus 4 others, ultimately covering almost 71,000 thyroid cancer survivors. The SIR for all SPC was a relatively modest 1.20, but the excess risk for selected, rarer cancers was notably higher (table 37).

For the most part, associations observed in the component studies have been confirmed in this meta-analysis. A notable exception is the absence of significant elevated risk for kidney cancer. As well, a protective effect for second cervical cancer was demonstrated, paralleling the pattern already seen for lung cancer. Again, low smoking rates in thyroid cancer patients may account for this phenomenon. Finally, the increased risk of second endocrine gland tumors was localized to the adrenal gland, as we have seen previously. We will briefly examine the SPC dynamic in this system of the body in the final subsection of this chapter.

To sum up our current topic, notwithstanding the open questions concerning the etiologic mechanism with specific SPC sites, the excess risk of many types of cancer following thyroid cancer, and the fact that thyroid cancer incidence is both growing and showing up in younger patients, suggests that the call for an intensive surveillance program related to SPC is prudent [107].

Table 37. SPC following thyroid cancer (pooled analysis)

SPC	Overall SIR
Lung	0.84 (0.75–0.92)
Colorectal	1.27 (1.13–1.41)
Colon	1.17 (1.05–1.28)
Breast	1.25 (1.17–1.32)
NHL	1.22 (1.03–1.42)
Brain	1.45 (1.12–1.78)
Prostate	1.38 (1.25–1.51)
Stomach	1.21 (1.02–1.40)
Leukemia	1.74 (1.46–2.02)
Multiple myeloma	1.33 (1.00–1.66)
Cervix	0.76 (0.57–0.95)
Soft tissue sarcoma	2.14 (1.46–2.83)
Salivary gland	2.97 (1.78–4.15)
Bone	3.04 (1.42–4.67)
Adrenal gland	6.54 (2.73–10.35)
All cancers	**1.20 (1.17–1.24)**

Figures in parentheses are 95% CI. Adapted from Subramanian et al. [123].

A Digression: SPC following Endocrine Gland Tumors

While not, strictly speaking, a head and neck topic, we offer here a set of data on SPCs following nonthyroid endocrine gland cancer (table 38) [46]. The most dramatic risk relates to second primaries located in the thyroid gland. Combined with the information gleaned about cancers following thyroid gland tumors, there is a strong suggestion of common carcinogenic risk factors at work in the endocrine system.

Ocular Melanoma

The investigation of SPC following ocular melanoma appears to be a relatively recent phenomenon. The evidence related to ocular melanoma as a first primary has been mixed and modest, with a 2004 Canadian study reporting no excess SPC risk [124]

Table 38. SPC following non-thyroid endocrine gland cancer by follow-up period

SPC	Overall SIR	Years of follow-up: SIR		
		<1 year	1–10 years	>10 years
Breast	1.2 (1.0–1.4)			
Kidney	2.6 (2.0–3.2)	14.3 (8.9–20.8)	1.7 (1.1–2.3)	2.5 (1.6–3.6)
Thyroid gland	9.2 (7.2–11.5)	121.6 (89.9–158.1)	3.1 (1.7–4.9)	
Other endocrine	3.5 (2.8–4.4)	20.8 (13.3–29.9)	2.3 (1.5–3.1)	3.2 (2.0–4.6)
Liver	1.5 (1.1–2.0)		1.6 (1.1–2.2)	
Small intestine	3.2 (1.7–5.1)	13.8 (2.6–33.9)	2.6 (1.0–4.9)	
Nervous system	2.7 (2.1–3.3)	13.3 (8.0–20.0)	2.0 (1.4–2.7)	2.2 (1.3–3.3)
All cancers	**1.3 (1.2–1.3)**	**3.8 (3.3–4.4)**	**1.1 (1.0–1.2)**	**1.2 (1.0–1.3)**

Figures in parentheses are 95% CI. Adapted from Hemminki and Jiang [46].

Table 39. SPC following ocular melanoma

SPC	Overall SIR
Pancreas	1.58 (1.16–2.11)
Prostate	1.31 (1.11–1.54)
Stomach	1.33 (1.03–1.68)
Kidney	1.70 (1.22–2.31)
Melanoma, skin	2.38 (1.77–3.14)
Multiple myeloma	2.00 (1.29–2.95)
Liver	3.89 (2.66–5.49)
All cancers	**1.24 (1.16–1.31)**

Figures in parentheses are 95% CI. Adapted from Scelo et al. [126].

and Swedish research suggesting an excess risk for all sites of only 13% (95% CI 1.02–1.26) [125] in 2006.

The best attempt to generate meaningful information involved a 2006 analysis of 13 population-based registries [126]. Table 39 presents the significant SIR data. The authors considered some of the associations to be artifacts of misclassification or (due to small absolute numbers) simply chance. It is possible that the elevated risk for prostate and kidney cancer may be due to common risk factors and mechanisms, possibly genetic in origin. The main discussion was reserved for the profile seen with second cutaneous melanomas. While melanomas occurring in the eye and skin are quite different cancers, they may share a common endogenous risk factor of genetic instability of melanocytes or an inability to repair DNA damage. Some of the apparently increased risk of cutaneous melanoma may be largely ascribed to more intensive follow-up (the so-called 'surveillance bias' or 'screening effect') rather than to common etiologic mechanisms.

Notes and References

1 This category usually comprises head and neck cancer, esophageal cancer and lung cancer. An alternate label sometimes employed for this collection of sites is respiratory and upper digestive tract (RUDT). We found 1 case where researchers considered lung and esophagus sites as additions to upper aerodigestive tract (generating the inelegant acronym UADT-E-L). The linkage between such sites again is etiological, specifically related to tobacco and alcohol consumption. Finally, we noted that sometimes researchers use head and neck and upper aerodigestive tract essentially as synonyms.

2 Tabor MP, Brakenhoff RH, Ruijter-Schippers HJ, et al: Multiple head and neck tumors frequently originate from a single preneoplastic lesion. Am J Pathol 2002;161:1051–1060.

3 Braakhuis BJ, Tabor MP, Leemans CR, et al: Second primary tumors and field cancerization in oral and oropharyngeal cancer: molecular techniques provide new insights and definitions. Head Neck 2002;24:198–206.

4 Giefing M, Rydzanicz M, Szukala K, et al: Second primary tumors (SPT) of head and neck: distinguishing of 'true' SPT from micrometastasis by LOH analysis of selected chromosome regions. Neoplasma 2005;52:374–380.

5 Braakhuis BJ, Tabor MP, Kummer JA, et al: A genetic explanation of Slaughter's concept of field cancerization: evidence and clinical implications. Cancer Res 2003;63:1727–1730.

6 Braakhuis BJ, Brakenhoff RH, Leemans CR: Second field tumors: a new opportunity for cancer prevention? Oncologist 2005;10:493–500.

7 Ronchetti D, Arisi E, Neri A, et al: Microsatellite analyses of recurrence or second primary tumor in head and neck cancer. Anticancer Res 2005;25: 2771–2775.

8 Van Oijen MG, Leppers vd Straat FG, Tilanus MG, et al: The origins of multiple squamous cell carcinomas in the aerodigestive tract. Cancer 2000;88:884–893.

9 Leong PP, Rezai B, Koch WM, et al: Distinguishing second primary tumors from lung metastases in patients with head and neck squamous cell carcinoma. J Natl Cancer Inst 1998;90:972–977.

10 Geurts TW, Nederlof PM, van den Brekel MW, et al: Pulmonary squamous cell carcinoma following head and neck squamous cell carcinoma: metastasis or second primary? Clin Cancer Res 2005;11:6608–6614.

11 Leon X, Ferlito A, Myer CM 3rd, et al: Second primary tumors in head and neck cancer patients. Acta Otolaryngol 2002;122:765–778.

12 Vaamonde P, Martin C, del Rio M, et al: Second primary malignancies in patients with cancer of the head and neck. Otolaryngol Head Neck Surg 2003; 129:65–70.

13 Warnakulasuriya KA, Robinson D, Evans H: Multiple primary tumours following head and neck cancer in southern England during 1961–98. J Oral Pathol Med 2003;32:443–449.

14 Ibid.

15 Specifically for tobacco-associated cancers.

16 Bhattacharyya N: An assessment of risk factors for the development of a second primary malignancy in the head and neck. Ear Nose Throat J 2006;85:121–125.

17 Deleyiannis FW, Thomas DB: Risk of lung cancer among patients with head and neck cancer. Otolaryngol Head Neck Surg 1997;116:630–636.

18 Argiris A, Brockstein BE, Haraf DJ, et al: Competing causes of death and second primary tumors in patients with locoregionally advanced head and neck cancer treated with chemoradiotherapy. Clin Cancer Res 2004;10:1956–1962.

19 Schwartz LH, Ozsahin M, Zhang GN, et al: Synchronous and metachronous head and neck carcinomas. Cancer 1994;74:1933–1938.

20 Note the confirming results in this regard in Do KA, Johnson MM, Lee JJ, et al: Longitudinal study of smoking patterns in relation to the development of smoking-related secondary primary tumors in patients with upper aerodigestive tract malignancies. Cancer 2004;101:2837–2842.

21 Garces YI, Schroeder DR, Nirelli LM, et al: Second primary tumors following tobacco dependence treatments among head and neck cancer patients. Am J Clin Oncol 2007;30:531–539.

22 Cited in Warnakulasuriya KA, Robinson D, Evans H: Multiple primary tumours following head and neck cancer in southern England during 1961–98. J Oral Pathol Med 2003;32:443–449.
23 Khuri FR, Kim ES, Lee JJ, et al: The impact of smoking status, disease stage, and index tumor site on second primary tumor incidence and tumor recurrence in the head and neck retinoid chemoprevention trial. Cancer Epidemiol Biomarkers Prev 2001; 10:823–829.
24 Tomek MS, McGuirt WF: Second head and neck cancers and tobacco usage. Am J Otolaryngol 2003; 24:24–27.
25 Parker RG, Enstrom JE: Second primary cancers of the head and neck following treatment of initial primary head and neck cancers. Int J Radiat Oncol Biol Phys 1988;14:561–564.
26 Munker R, Purmale L, Aydemir U, et al: Advanced head and neck cancer: long-term results of chemoradiotherapy, complications and induction of second malignancies. Onkologie 2001;24:553–558.
27 Taussky D, Rufibach K, Huguenin P, et al: Risk factors for developing a second upper aerodigestive cancer after radiotherapy with or without chemotherapy in patients with head-and-neck cancers: an exploratory outcomes analysis. Int J Radiat Oncol Biol Phys 2005;62:684–689.
28 Amemiya K, Shibuya H, Yoshimura R, et al: The risk of radiation-induced cancer in patients with squamous cell carcinoma of the head and neck and its results of treatment. Br J Radiol 2005;78: 1028–1033.
29 Demirkan F, Unal S, Cenetoglu S, et al: Radiation-induced leiomyosarcomas as second primary tumors in the head and neck region: report of 2 cases. J Oral Maxillofac Surg 2003;61:259–263.
30 Bongers V, Braakhuis BJ, Tobi H, et al: The relation between cancer incidence among relatives and the occurrence of multiple primary carcinomas following head and neck cancer. Cancer Epidemiol Biomarkers Prev 1996;5:595–598.
31 Llewellyn CD, Johnson NW, Warnakulasuriya KA: Risk factors for squamous cell carcinoma of the oral cavity in young people – a comprehensive literature review. Oral Oncol 2001;37:401–418.
32 Jefferies S, Foulkes WD: Genetic mechanisms in squamous cell carcinoma of the head and neck. Oral Oncol 2001;37:115–126.
33 Muto M, Takahashi M, Ohtsu A, et al: Risk of multiple squamous cell carcinomas both in the esophagus and the head and neck region. Carcinogenesis 2005;26:1008–1012.
34 Klaassen I, Braakhuis BJ: Anticancer activity and mechanism of action of retinoids in oral and pharyngeal cancer. Oral Oncol 2002;38:532–542.
35 Schwartz JL: Biomarkers and molecular epidemiology and chemoprevention of oral carcinogenesis. Crit Rev Oral Biol Med 2000;11:92–122.
36 Mayne ST, Cartmel B, Baum M, et al: Randomized trial of supplemental β-carotene to prevent second head and neck cancer. Cancer Res 2001;61: 1457–1463.
37 Van Zandwijk N, Dalesio O, Pastorino U, et al: EUROSCAN, a randomized trial of vitamin A and N-acetylcysteine in patients with head and neck cancer or lung cancer. For the European Organization for Research and Treatment of Cancer Head and Neck and Lung Cancer Cooperative Groups. J Natl Cancer Inst 2000;92:977–986.
38 Kim ES, Hong WK, Khuri FR: Chemoprevention of aerodigestive tract cancers. Ann Rev Med 2002;53: 223–243.
39 Choe MS, Zhang X, Shin HJ, et al: Interaction between epidermal growth factor receptor- and cyclooxygenase 2-mediated pathways and its implications for the chemoprevention of head and neck cancer. Mol Cancer Ther 2005;4:1448–1455.
40 Khuri FR, Lee JJ, Lippman SM, et al: Randomized phase III trial of low-dose isotretinoin for prevention of second primary tumors in stage I and II head and neck cancer patients. J Natl Cancer Inst 2006; 98:441–450.
41 Perry CF, Stevens M, Rabie I, et al: Chemoprevention of head and neck cancer with retinoids: a negative result. Arch Otolaryngol Head Neck Surg 2005;131:198–203.
42 Bairati I, Meyer F, Gelinas M, et al: A randomized trial of antioxidant vitamins to prevent second primary cancers in head and neck cancer patients. J Natl Cancer Inst 2005;97:481–488.
43 Venuti A, Manni V, Morello R, et al: Physical state and expression of human papillomavirus in laryngeal carcinoma and surrounding normal mucosa. J Med Virol 2000;60:396–402.
44 Major T, Szarka K, Sziklai I, et al: The characteristics of human papillomavirus DNA in head and neck cancers and papillomas. J Clin Pathol 2005;58:51–55.
45 Gillison ML, Shah KV: Chapter 9: role of mucosal human papillomavirus in nongenital cancers. J Natl Cancer Inst Monogr 2003;31:57–65.
46 Hemminki K, Jiang Y, Dong C: Second primary cancers after anogenital, skin, oral, esophageal and rectal cancers: etiological links? Int J Cancer 2001; 93:294–298.
47 Rodrigues VC, Moss SM, Tuomainen H: Oral cancer in the UK: to screen or not to screen. Oral Oncol 1998;34:454–465.
48 Yamamoto E, Shibuya H, Yoshimura R, et al: Site specific dependency of second primary cancer in early stage head and neck squamous cell carcinoma. Cancer 2002;94:2007–2014.

49 Sood S, Bradley PJ, Quraishi S: Second primary tumors in squamous cell carcinoma of the head and neck – incidence, site, location, and prevention. Curr Opin Otolaryngol Head Neck Surg 2000;8: 87–90.
50 Wu X, Zhao H, Do KA, et al: Serum levels of insulin growth factor (IGF-I) and IGF-binding protein predict risk of second primary tumors in patients with head and neck cancer. Clin Cancer Res 2004;10: 3988–3995.
51 Cloos J, Leemans CR, van der Sterre ML, et al: Mutagen sensitivity as a biomarker for second primary tumors after head and neck squamous cell carcinoma. Cancer Epidemiol Biomarkers Prev 2000;9:713–717.
52 See Neugut AI, Meadows AT, Robinson E (eds): Multiple Primary Cancers. Philadelphia, Lippincott Williams & Wilkins, 1999. The relevant chapter in *Multiple Primary Cancers* follows this pattern, covering head and neck, lung as well as esophageal cancers under the broad heading of the upper aerodigestive tract. The inclusion of the lung can be confusing, as it sometimes is differentiated from the oropharynx by being classified as part of the lower respiratory tract.
53 Li X, Hemminki K: Familial upper aerodigestive tract cancers: incidence trends, familial clustering and subsequent cancers. Oral Oncol 2003;39: 232–239.
54 Other than ovaries and uterus.
55 Do KA, Johnson MM, Doherty DA, et al: Second primary tumors in patients with upper aerodigestive tract cancers: joint effects of smoking and alcohol (United States). Cancer Causes Control 2003; 14:131–138.
56 Morita M, Saeki H, Mori M, et al: Risk factors for esophageal cancer and the multiple occurrence of carcinoma in the upper aerodigestive tract. Surgery 2002;131(suppl):S1–S6.
57 Smith W, Saba N: Retinoids as chemoprevention for head and neck cancer: where do we go from here? Crit Rev Oncol Hematol 2005;55:143–152.
58 Anderson WF, Hawk E, Berg CD: Secondary chemoprevention of upper aerodigestive tract tumors. Semin Oncol 2001;28:106–120.
59 Xu H, Lu DW, El-Mofty SK, et al: Metachronous squamous cell carcinomas evolving from independent oropharyngeal and pulmonary squamous papillomas: association with human papillomavirus 11 and lack of aberrant p53, Rb, and p16 protein expression. Hum Pathol 2004;35:1419–1422.
60 Some studies also amalgamate the esophagus and the hypopharynx.
61 Kramer FJ, Janssen M, Eckardt A: Second primary tumours in oropharyngeal squamous cell carcinoma. Clin Oral Invest 2004;8:56–62.
62 Crosher R, McIlroy R: The incidence of other primary tumours in patients with oral cancer in Scotland. Br J Oral Maxillofac Surg 1998;36:58–62.
63 McDowell JD: An overview of epidemiology and common risk factors for oral squamous cell carcinoma. Otolaryngol Clin North Am 2006;39: 277–294.
64 Soderholm AL, Pukkala E, Lindqvist C, et al: Risk of new primary cancer in patients with oropharyngeal cancer. Br J Cancer 1994;69:784–787.
65 Shibuya H, Wakita T, Nakagawa T, et al: The relation between an esophageal cancer and associated cancers in adjacent organs. Cancer 1995;76:101–105.
66 Day GL, Blot WJ: Second primary tumors in patients with oral cancer. Cancer 1992;70:14–19.
67 Schou G, Storm HH, Jensen OM: Second cancer following cancers of the buccal cavity and pharynx in Denmark, 1943–80. Natl Cancer Inst Monogr 1985; 68:253–276.
68 Lissowska J, Pilarska A, Pilarski P, et al: Smoking, alcohol, diet, dentition and sexual practices in the epidemiology of oral cancer in Poland. Eur J Cancer Prev 2003;12:25–33.
69 Day GL, Shore RE, Blot WJ, et al: Dietary factors and second primary cancers: a follow-up of oral and pharyngeal cancer patients. Nutr Cancer 1994;21:223–232.
70 Bolla M, Lefur R, Ton Van J, et al: Prevention of second primary tumours with etretinate in squamous cell carcinoma of the oral cavity and oropharynx: results of a multicentric double-blind randomised study. Eur J Cancer 1994;30A:767–772.
71 Hashibe M, Ritz B, Le AD, et al: Radiotherapy for oral cancer as a risk factor for second primary cancers. Cancer Lett 2005;220:185–195.
72 Kishino M, Shibuya H, Yoshimura R, et al: A retrospective analysis of the use of brachytherapy in relation to early stage squamous cell carcinoma of the oropharynx and its relationship to second primary respiratory and upper digestive tract cancers. Br J Radiol 2007;80:121–125.
73 Day GL, Blot WJ, Shore RE, et al: Second cancers following oral and pharyngeal cancers: role of tobacco and alcohol. J Natl Cancer Inst 1994;86: 131–137.
74 Van der Tol IG, de Visscher JG, Jovanovic A, et al: Risk of second primary cancer following treatment of squamous cell carcinoma of the lower lip. Oral Oncol 1999;35:571–574.
75 Shibuya H, Amagasa T, Seto K, et al: Leukoplakia-associated multiple carcinomas in patients with tongue carcinoma. Cancer 1986;57:843–846.
76 Sessions DG, Lenox J, Spector GJ, et al: Analysis of treatment results for base of tongue cancer. Laryngoscope 2003;113:1252–1261.

77 Mizobuchi S, Kato H, Tachimori Y, et al: Multiple primary carcinoma of the oesophagus. Surg Oncol 1993;2:249–253.

78 Sun EC, Curtis R, Melbye M, et al: Salivary gland cancer in the United States. Cancer Epidemiol Biomarkers Prev 1999;8:1095–1100.

79 In der Maur CD, Klokman WJ, van Leeuwen FE, et al: Increased risk of breast cancer development after diagnosis of salivary gland tumour. Eur J Cancer 2005; 41:1311–1315.

80 Ibid.

81 Ramos-Casals M, Loustaud-Ratti V, De Vita S, et al: Sjogren syndrome associated with hepatitis C virus: a multicenter analysis of 137 cases. Medicine 2005;84:81–89.

82 Sham JS, Wei WI, Tai PT, et al: Multiple malignant neoplasms in patients with nasopharyngeal carcinoma. Oncology 1990;47:471–474.

83 Teshima T, Inoue T, Chatani M, et al: Incidence of other primary cancers in 1,569 patients with pharyngolaryngeal cancer and treated with radiation therapy. Strahlenther Onkol 1992;168:213–218.

84 Chen CL, Hsu MM: Second primary epithelial malignancy of nasopharynx and nasal cavity after successful curative radiation therapy of nasopharyngeal carcinoma. Hum Pathol 2000;31:227–232.

85 Wang CC, Chen ML, Hsu KH, et al: Second malignant tumors in patients with nasopharyngeal carcinoma and their association with Epstein-Barr virus. Int J Cancer 2000;87:228–231.

86 This overall SIR figure applies to both lymphoma and leukemia.

87 Scelo G, Boffetta P, Corbex M, et al: Second primary cancers in patients with nasopharyngeal carcinoma: a pooled analysis of 13 cancer registries. Cancer Causes Control 2007;18:269–278.

88 Teo PM, Chan AT, Leung SF, et al: Increased incidence of tongue cancer after primary radiotherapy for nasopharyngeal carcinoma – the possibility of radiation carcinogenesis. Eur J Cancer 1999;35:219–225.

89 Gao X, Fisher SG, Mohideen N, et al: Second primary cancers in patients with laryngeal cancer: a population-based study. Int J Radiat Oncol Biol Phys 2003;56:427–435.

90 Levi F, Randimbison L, Te VC, et al: Second primary cancers in laryngeal cancer patients. Eur J Cancer 2003;39:265–267.

91 Sjogren EV, Snijder S, van Beekum J, et al: Second malignant neoplasia in early (TIS-T1) glottic carcinoma. Head Neck 2006;28:501–507.

92 Ecimovic P, Pompe-Kirn V: Second primary cancers in laryngeal cancer patients in Slovenia, 1961–1996. Eur J Cancer 2002;38:1254–1260.

93 Albright JT, Karpati R, Topham AK, et al: Second malignant neoplasms in patients under 40 years of age with laryngeal cancer. Laryngoscope 2001;111: 563–567.

94 Schwager K, Nebel A, Baier G, et al: Second primary carcinomas in the upper aerodigestive tract in different locations and age groups. Laryngorhinootologie 2000;79:599–603.

95 Natsugoe S, Matsumoto M, Okumura H, et al: Multiple primary carcinomas with esophageal squamous cell cancer: clinicopathologic outcome. World J Surg 2005;29:46–49.

96 Kumagai Y, Kawano T, Nakajima Y, et al: Multiple primary cancers associated with esophageal carcinoma. Surg Today 2001;31:872–876.

97 Wu X, Hu Y, Lippman SM: Upper aerodigestive tract cancers; in Neugut AI, Meadows AT, Robinson E (eds): Multiple Primary Cancers. Philadelphia, Lippincott Williams & Wilkins, 1999.

98 Nagasawa S, Onda M, Sasajima K, et al: Multiple primary malignant neoplasms in patients with esophageal cancer. Dis Esophagus 2000;13:226–230.

99 Morita M, Saeki H, Mori M, et al: Risk factors for esophageal cancer and the multiple occurrence of carcinoma in the upper aerodigestive tract. Surgery 2002;131(suppl):S1–S6.

100 Levi F, Randimbison L, Maspoli M, et al: Second neoplasms after oesophageal cancer. Int J Cancer 2007;121:694–697.

101 Poon RT, Law SY, Chu KM, et al: Multiple primary cancers in esophageal squamous cell carcinoma: incidence and implications. Ann Thorac Surg 1998; 65:1529–1534.

102 Noguchi T, Kato T, Takeno S, et al: Necessity of screening for multiple primary cancers in patients with esophageal cancer. Ann Thorac Cardiovasc Surg 2002;8:336–342.

103 Motoyama S, Saito R, Kitamura M, et al: Outcomes of active operation during intensive followup for second primary malignancy after esophagectomy for thoracic squamous cell esophageal carcinoma. J Am Coll Surg 2003;197:914–920.

104 Salminen EK, Pukkala E, Kiel KD, et al: Impact of radiotherapy in the risk of esophageal cancer as subsequent primary cancer after breast cancer. Int J Radiat Oncol Biol Phys 2006;65:699–704.

105 Ronckers CM, McCarron P, Ron E: Thyroid cancer and multiple primary tumors in the SEER cancer registries. Int J Cancer 2005;117:281–288.

106 Mack WJ, Preston-Martin S, Dal Maso L, et al: A pooled analysis of case-control studies of thyroid cancer: cigarette smoking and consumption of alcohol, coffee, and tea. Cancer Causes Control 2003;14: 773–785.

107 Sandeep TC, Strachan MW, Reynolds RM, et al: Second primary cancers in thyroid cancer patients: a multinational record linkage study. J Clin Endocrinol Metab 2006;91:1819–1825.

108 Excluding thyroid.

109 Excluding thyroid.

110 Berthe E, Henry-Amar M, Michels JJ, et al: Risk of second primary cancer following differentiated thyroid cancer. Eur J Nucl Med Mol Imaging 2004;31:685–691.
111 Canchola AJ, Horn-Ross PL, Purdie DM: Risk of second primary malignancies in women with papillary thyroid cancer. Am J Epidemiol 2006;163:521–527.
112 Rubino C, de Vathaire F, Dottorini ME, et al: Second primary malignancies in thyroid cancer patients. Br J Cancer 2003;89:1638–1644.
113 On I-131 and colorectal cancer, note the strong support in de Vathaire F, Schlumberger M, Delisle MJ, et al: Leukaemias and cancers following iodine-131 administration for thyroid cancer. Br J Cancer 1997;75:734–739.
114 Chuang SC, Hashibe M, Yu GP, et al: Radiotherapy for primary thyroid cancer as a risk factor for second primary cancers. Cancer Lett 2006;238:42–52.
115 Bhattacharyya N, Chien W: Risk of second primary malignancy after radioactive iodine treatment for differentiated thyroid carcinoma. Ann Otol Rhinol Laryngol 2006;115:607–610.
116 Verkooijen RB, Smit JW, Romijn JA, et al: The incidence of second primary tumors in thyroid cancer patients is increased, but not related to treatment of thyroid cancer. Eur J Endocrinol 2006;155:801–806.
117 Adjadj E, Rubino C, Shamsaldim A, et al: The risk of multiple primary breast and thyroid carcinomas. Cancer 2003;98:1309–1317.
118 Sadetzki S, Calderon-Margalit R, Peretz C, et al: Second primary breast and thyroid cancers (Israel). Cancer Causes Control 2003;14:367–375.
119 Li CI, Rossing MA, Voigt LF, et al: Multiple primary breast and thyroid cancers: role of age at diagnosis and cancer treatments (United States). Cancer Causes Control 2000;11:805–811.
120 Cristofanilli M, Yamamura Y, Kau SW, et al: Thyroid hormone and breast carcinoma: primary hypothyroidism is associated with a reduced incidence of primary breast carcinoma. Cancer 2005;103:1122–1128.
121 Vassilopoulou-Sellin R, Palmer L, Taylor S, et al: Incidence of breast carcinoma in women with thyroid carcinoma. Cancer 1999;85:696–705.
122 Chen AY, Levy L, Goepfert H, et al: The development of breast carcinoma in women with thyroid carcinoma. Cancer 2001;92:225–231.
123 Subramanian S, Goldstein DP, Parlea L, et al: Second primary malignancy risk in thyroid cancer survivors: a systematic review and meta-analysis. Thyroid 2007;17:1277–1288.
124 Callejo SA, Al-Khalifa S, Ozdal PC, et al: The risk of other primary cancer in patients with uveal melanoma: a retrospective cohort study of a Canadian population. Can J Ophthalmol 2004;39:397–402.
125 Bergman L, Nilsson B, Ragnarsson-Olding B, et al: Uveal melanoma: a study on incidence of additional cancers in the Swedish population. Invest Ophthalmol Vis Sci 2006;47:72–77.
126 Scelo G, Boffetta P, Autier P, et al: Associations between ocular melanoma and other primary cancers: an international population-based study. Int J Cancer 2007;120:152–159.

Krueger H, McLean D, Williams D: The Prevention of Second Primary Cancers.
Prog Exp Tumor Res. Basel, Karger, 2008, vol 40, pp 85–91

10

Gastrointestinal Cancers

In this chapter, we will consider SPC following cancer of the stomach, pancreas, liver, gall bladder and related ducts, small intestine as well as large intestine (that is, colon and rectum). The most extensive research has occurred in the case of the latter category, usually under the heading of colorectal cancer. The strongest associations following cancer of the gastrointestinal tract are usually related to second primaries in the gastrointestinal tract itself [1]. For instance, the few studies available reveal that cancer of the gall bladder is linked to a higher incidence of colonic and gastric carcinomas [2–4].

Stomach

We have already covered the mouth and esophagus in the preceding chapter. So, turning to the next part of the gastrointestinal tract, the stomach, the first important observation is that associations between gastric cancer and SPC 'are not so clear-cut as for other tumors' [5]. The site most often connected to an elevated risk of SPC is the stomach itself, followed by the colon, liver and lung [6]. Despite the lung being on this list, gastric cancer has not generally been connected with tobacco-related malignancies (see the relationship to smoking noted below). The only significant risk identified in the *Multiple Primary Cancers* monograph related to the SIR of 2.2 for a second primary lymphoma following gastric cancer [7]. Research since that text was published has not appreciably extended the knowledge base; the gaps may be partly related to the high mortality with stomach cancer – patients simply may not have the time to develop a clear SPC profile. Nonetheless, some researchers have reinforced the importance of surveillance for SPC following early gastric cancer [8–10]. Other papers have added 2 other suggestions:

(1) breast cancer should be on the watch list of suspected sites for SPC (despite the fact that no clear evidence of excess risk has yet been developed) [11];
(2) among males, smokers experience almost twice the risk for SPC compared with nonsmokers [12].

Table 40. SPC following cancer of the small intestine

SPC	Overall SIR
Colon	3.41 (2.40–4.70)
Rectum	3.17 (1.96–4.84)
Pancreas	2.75 (1.42–4.80)
Ovary	4.12 (1.98–7.58)
Gall bladder	4.64 (1.87–9.56)
Soft tissue sarcoma	5.15 (1.06–15.00)
Non-melanoma skin cancer	1.91 (1.09–3.11)
All cancers	**1.68 (1.47–1.91)**

Figures in parentheses are 95% CI. Adapted from Scelo et al. [14].

Pancreas, Liver and Gallbladder

From the stomach, we can quickly pass to the small intestine. This is because, following the pattern seen in other deadly cancers (such as the esophageal variety), there are few data for SPC following pancreatic or liver cancer. The limited results available for the gallbladder (and related ducts) were noted above. The simple fact is that patients with such malignancies rarely survive long enough to develop or detect a second primary. When information is produced, it does not allow for an accurate assessment of excess risks for SPC [13].

Small Intestine

In contrast to the preceding categories, a large 2006 study conducted by Scelo et al. [14] examined almost 11,000 cases of small intestine cancer and found strongly elevated risks for several SPCs (table 40).

An earlier, smaller study showed an association with colorectal cancer, and also suggested excess risks for skin melanoma and prostate cancer, though the data were specific to certain cell types [15]. The discussion concerning excess colorectal cancer has centered on shared genetic pathways, including the hereditary nonpolyposis colorectal cancer syndrome [16]. Many of the associations with small intestine cancer remain obscure in origin, though shared risk factors and mechanisms are suspected. One of the most intriguing suggestions with respect to intestinal and oropharyngeal

Table 41. SPC following carcinoid tumors of the small intestine

SPC	Overall SIR
Oropharynx	5.77 (1.19–16.9)
Thyroid gland	3.33 (1.08–7.77)
Nonmelanoma skin cancer	2.12 (1.39–3.11)
All cancers	**1.18 (1.05–1.32)**

Figures in parentheses are 95% CI. Adapted from Scelo et al. [14].

cancer associations relates to the common effect of chronic inflammatory conditions such as Crohn's or celiac disease [14].

An illustration of stratification by tissue category was also provided in the research of Scelo and colleagues. It examined the risk of SPC specifically following carcinoid [17] of the small intestine. In table 41, it is clear that the data deviate from that of small intestine cancer as a whole. Several SPCs have been dropped from the list, while oropharyngeal and thyroid gland cancers have been added.

It is not clear whether the emerging risk profiles related to the aggregate and specific tissues of the small intestine can lead to anything other than a secondary prevention program involving targeted surveillance.

Finally, on our journey through the gastrointestinal tract, we come to the large intestine, and to the consequences of primary colorectal tumors.

Colorectal Cancer

As noted above, the investigation of SPC has been most thorough with respect to a first primary cancer of the colorectum. The largest study (by a wide margin) was based on 217,705 patients in the US SEER database. While the published information did not detail results for specific SPCs, it did confirm a significant and precise excess risk following colorectal cancer (SIR = 1.9, 95% CI 1.8–1.9) [18].

The next most extensive study involved the examination of 127,281 patients in England [19]. Table 42 presents the significant data for those with a colorectal cancer diagnosis before the age of 60 years (in men) and 65 years (in women).

The first observation is that the colorectum is one of those sites, like the breast and the lung, where multiple primaries are common. Indeed, the phenomenon of multiple primaries arising in the colorectum generally appears to dominate the SPC story [20]. Outside the index site, significant data are limited to the eye (in men) and

Table 42. SPC following colorectal cancer

SPC	Overall SIR	
	men <60 years	women <65 years
Colon	2.33 (1.81–2.95)	1.28 (1.02–1.60)
Ovary		2.56 (2.11–3.09)
Cervix		1.61 (1.12–2.24)
Uterus		1.56 (1.18–2.02)
Eye	4.03 (1.31–9.41)	
All cancers	**1.09 (1.00–1.20)**	**1.19 (1.11–1.28)**

Figures in parentheses are 95% CI. Adapted from Evans et al. [19].

Table 43. SPC following colorectal cancer by follow-up period

SPC	Years of follow-up: SIR		
	<1 year	1–10 years	>10 years
Upper aerodigestive tract		1.35 (1.07–1.66)	1.56 (1.06–2.16)
Colorectum	2.70 (2.25–3.20)	2.03 (1.88–2.19)	2.40 (2.14–2.68)
Different subsites	3.03 (2.49–3.63)	2.21 (2.22–2.60)	2.68 (2.39–3.00)
Female breast	1.59 (1.18–2.07)	1.23 (1.09–1.38)	
Pancreas	2.12 (1.38–3.01)		1.46 (1.08–1.90)
NHL	2.12 (1.37–3.04)		
Ovary	7.39 (5.43–9.65)	1.68 (1.33–2.07)	
Prostate	2.51 (2.16–2.90)	1.22 (1.12–1.32)	1.20 (1.05–1.37)
Leukemia	2.20 (1.38–3.22)		
Stomach	2.22 (1.61–2.94)		
Kidney	4.48 (3.36–5.77)	1.56 (1.30–1.84)	
Urinary bladder	1.76 (1.23–2.38)	1.34 (1.15–1.53)	
Melanoma, skin	2.20 (1.28–3.37)	1.67 (1.34–2.03)	
Cervix	2.71 (1.23–4.77)		
Other female genitals		2.11 (1.32–3.09)	
Endometrium	2.08 (1.19–3.22)	1.87 (1.53–2.24)	1.64 (1.16–2.21)
Other male genitals			3.75 (1.35–7.35)
Thyroid gland	3.88 (1.66–7.04)		2.74 (1.53–4.29)
Liver	2.41 (1.62–3.35)		
Small intestine	33.96 (25.58–43.53)	3.91 (2.85–5.14)	2.35 (1.12–4.02)
Endocrine gland	3.20 (1.82–4.96)	1.37 (1.01–1.78)	
Nervous system	2.95 (1.89–4.25)		
Nonmelanoma skin cancer		1.23 (1.03–1.44)	
All cancers	**2.33 (2.18–2.49)**	**1.33 (1.28–1.37)**	**1.37 (1.30–1.44)**

Figures in parentheses are 95% CI. Adapted from Hemminki et al. [21].

gynecological cancers. While the cervix and uterus may well be within the radiation field in some female patients, the ocular association is difficult to explain, as is its restriction to males.

A 2001 Swedish study of about 68,000 cases of colorectal cancer revealed even a wider range of implicated SPCs, especially for cases diagnosed in the first year (table 43) [21]. It is important to note that such results may reflect, in part, the effect of common genetic or other factors, or simply bias due to intensified surveillance.

Aside from confirming the excess risk of colorectal and uterine cancers, this study added the upper aerodigestive tract, pancreas, prostate and other male genital organs, thyroid gland as well as the small intestine as sites demonstrating long-term concern regarding cancer development. Several of these SPCs may be a reflection of common genetic risks, for example, related to the hereditary nonpolyposis colorectal cancer syndrome mentioned above [22]. The latter disorder certainly is one of the drivers of multiple primaries localized in the colorectum itself, as well as the excess risk seen in SPC of the small intestine.

The topic of multiple primary colorectal cancer of both synchronous and metachronous varieties is a specialized study of its own, and one that, by our definition of SPC, technically lies outside the scope of this monograph. It will suffice to note here that, even after controlling for familial patterns, metachronous colorectal cancer still occurs at a higher rate than first primaries in the general population. Genetic factors other than hereditary nonpolyposis colorectal cancer syndrome have been implicated in this phenomenon [23, 24]. A helpful result from the 2001 Swedish study is that an excess risk of 'true' SPC (that is, outside the colorectum) applies even when familial patterns are controlled. The significant SIR for second cancers following so-called sporadic (that is, nonfamilial) colorectal cancer was 2.16, compared to 6.46 in cases of familial colorectal cancer [22]. Clearly, when there is evidence of familial cancer, and especially if there is definite molecular corroboration by gene testing, surveillance is particularly important. This would pertain in particular to gynecological cancers [25].

When posited genetic factors are not reasonably able to account for all the excess risk, we must turn to therapy effects or environmental causes. The standard treatment for colorectal cancer is surgery, sometimes with adjuvant radio- or chemotherapy. Again, the Swedish data noted earlier suggest that any therapy effect following colorectal cancer is not large, as the various SPC risks often declined rather than increased with time (table 43) [26]. A 2005 study offered another view of any complications following radiotherapy, stressing the need to pursue radiation treatment, based on 'the reduced risk of the sum of local recurrences and second cancers' [27]. In other words, there is a net gain attached to radiotherapy.

A 2006 study was also reassuring about radiation for rectal cancer, pointing out that second cancers in adjacent tissues seemed to be reduced in frequency [28]. The researchers hypothesized that this effect could be attributed to some of the 'nascent but quiescent' tumors in, for instance, the prostate gland actually being cured by spillover irradiation from the rectal cancer therapy. A similar effect may be seen in any accidental ovarian ablation that would then lead to reduced (hormonally related) breast cancer rates. The authors further explain that the still elevated rates of uterine cancer (of both cervix and corpus) seen with adjacent radiation are due to the lower 'background frequency' of cancer in these tissues, especially compared with the prostate. In other words, any excess cancers show up more easily, and there are fewer nascent cancers to be incidentally 'cured' by radiotherapy for rectal cancer. Whatever the validity of this subtle argument, the simple epidemiologic conclusion is that therapy for rectal cancer does not seem to yield much explanatory power to account for any excess SPCs.

Finally, some of the excess cancers related specifically to anogenital squamous cell epithelia may be traceable to well-known environmental risk factors such as tobacco use and HPV infection [22, 29]. These potentially modifiable factors notwithstanding, the bottom line concerning SPCs in colorectal cancer patients has to involve a focus on surveillance and secondary prevention [30].

Notes and References

1 Watanabe S, Kodama T, Shimosato Y, et al: Second primary cancers in patients with gastrointestinal cancers. Jpn J Clin Oncol 1985;15(suppl 1):171–182.

2 Kamisawa T, Egawa N, Tsuruta K, et al: An investigation of primary malignancies associated with ampullary carcinoma. Hepatogastroenterology 2005;52: 22–24.

3 Das A, Neugut AI, Cooper GS, et al: Association of ampullary and colorectal malignancies. Cancer 2004; 100:524–530.

4 Nakamura S, Suzuki S, Sakaguchi T, et al: Second cancer during long-term survival after resection of biliary tract carcinoma. J Gastroenterol 1996;31: 289–293.

5 Neugut AI, Gold D: Gastrointestinal cancers; in Neugut AI, Meadows AT, Robinson E (eds): Multiple Primary Cancers. Philadelphia, Lippincott Williams & Wilkins, 1999.

6 Ikeguchi M, Ohfuji S, Oka A, et al: Synchronous and metachronous primary malignancies in organs other than the stomach in patients with early gastric cancer. Hepatogastroenterology 1995;42:672–676.

7 Neugut AI, Meadows AT, Robinson E (eds): Multiple Primary Cancers. Philadelphia, Lippincott Williams & Wilkins, 1999.

8 Ikeda Y, Saku M, Kawanaka H, et al: Features of second primary cancer in patients with gastric cancer. Oncology 2003;65:113–117.

9 Muela Molinero A, Jorquera Plaza F, Ribas Arino T, et al: Multiple malignant primary neoplasms in patients with gatric neoplasms in the health district of Leon. Rev Esp Enferm Dig 2006;98:907–916.

10 Ikeda Y, Saku M, Kishihara F, et al: Effective follow-up for recurrence or a second primary cancer in patients with early gastric cancer. Br J Surg 2005;92: 235–239.

11 Dinis-Ribeiro M, Lomba-Viana H, Silva R, et al: Associated primary tumors in patients with gastric cancer. J Clin Gastroenterol 2002;34:533–535.

12 Kinoshita Y, Tsukuma H, Ajiki W, et al: The risk for second primaries in gastric cancer patients: adjuvant therapy and habitual smoking and drinking. J Epidemiol 2000;10:300–304.

13 Wong LL, Lurie F, Takanishi DM Jr: Other primary neoplasms in patients with hepatocellular cancer: prognostic implications? Hawaii Med J 2007;66:204, 206–208.

14 Scelo G, Boffetta P, Hemminki K, et al: Associations between small intestine cancer and other primary cancers: an international population-based study. Int J Cancer 2006;118:189–196.

15 Neugut AI, Santos J: The association between cancers of the small and large bowel. Cancer Epidemiol Biomarkers Prev 1993;2:551–553.

16 Ripley D, Weinerman BH: Increased incidence of second malignancies associated with small bowel adenocarcinoma. Can J Gastroenterol 1997;11:65–68.

17 Carcinoid tumors arise from neuroendocrine cells and may develop in almost any organ. The most common gastrointestinal site is not the appendix (as is often quoted), but the small intestine, followed in frequency by the rectum. See Maggard MA, O'Connell JB, Ko CY: Updated population-based review of carcinoid tumors. Ann Surg 2004;240: 117–122. On the incidence of SPC following carcinoid tumors, see Rivadeneira DE, Tuckson WB, Naab T: Increased incidence of second primary malignancy in patients with carcinoid tumors: case report and literature review. J Natl Med Assoc 1996;88: 310–312. In chapter 8 (pp 56–61), we also looked at the SPC profile following carconoid tumors of the lung.
18 Shureiqi I, Cooksley CD, Morris J, et al: Effect of age on risk of second primary colorectal cancer. J Natl Cancer Inst 2001;93:1264–1266.
19 Evans HS, Moller H, Robinson D, et al: The risk of subsequent primary cancers after colorectal cancer in southeast England. Gut 2002;50:647–652.
20 Das A, Chak A, Cooper GS: Temporal trend in relative risk of second primary colorectal cancer. Am J Gastroenterol 2006;101:1342–1347.
21 Hemminki K, Li X, Dong C: Second primary cancers after sporadic and familial colorectal cancer. Cancer Epidemiol Biomarkers Prev 2001;10:793–798.
22 Hemminki K, Chen B: Familial association of colorectal adenocarcinoma with cancers at other sites. Eur J Cancer 2004;40:2480–2487.
23 Park IJ, Yu CS, Kim HC, et al: Metachronous colorectal cancer. Colorectal Dis 2006;8:323–327.
24 Sengupta SB, Yiu CY, Boulos PB, et al: Genetic instability in patients with metachronous colorectal cancers. Br J Surg 1997;84:996–1000.
25 Lu KH, Dinh M, Kohlmann W, et al: Gynecologic cancer as a 'sentinel cancer' for women with hereditary nonpolyposis colorectal cancer syndrome. Obstet Gynecol 2005;105:569–574.
26 Also note the trial described in Wolmark N, Wieand HS, Hyams DM, et al: Randomized trial of postoperative adjuvant chemotherapy with or without radiotherapy for carcinoma of the rectum: National Surgical Adjuvant Breast and Bowel Project Protocol R-02. J Natl Cancer Inst 2000;92:388–396.
27 Birgisson H, Pahlman L, Gunnarsson U, et al: Occurrence of second cancers in patients treated with radiotherapy for rectal cancer. J Clin Oncol 2005;23: 6126–6131.
28 Kendal WS, Nicholas G: A population-based analysis of second primary cancers after irradiation for rectal cancer. Am J Clin Oncol 2007;30:333–339.
29 Hemminki K, Jiang Y, Dong C: Second primary cancers after anogenital, skin, oral, esophageal and rectal cancers: etiological links? Int J Cancer 2001; 93:294–298.
30 Chiang JM, Yeh CY, Changehien CR, et al: Clinical features of second other-site primary cancers among sporadic colorectal cancer patients – a hospital-based study of 3,722 cases. Hepatogastroenterology 2004;51: 1341–1344.

Krueger H, McLean D, Williams D: The Prevention of Second Primary Cancers.
Prog Exp Tumor Res. Basel, Karger, 2008, vol 40, pp 92–101

11

Genitourinary Cancers

Before covering male-specific sites such as the prostate and the testes, we will address a topic common to both genders, namely, SPC following urological malignancies.

Kidney

The literature regarding SPC following urological cancers is limited. The main sites of interest include the kidney, the upper urinary tract in general and the bladder. Regarding kidney cancer, the 2 most recent studies were based on a similar sample size. In 2006, Beisland et al. [1] investigated 1,425 patients with renal cell carcinoma. Only 3 types of SPC showed a significant excess risk (table 44).

The results support the common understanding of bladder cancer as a key sequela to renal cancer. For instance, Rabbani and colleagues found that only bladder cancer was seen to exhibit an excess risk among a small series of renal carcinoma patients [2]. The common risk factor posited to explain this phenomenon involves smoking-related carcinogens excreted through the kidneys and thence to the bladder and its tissues [3].

The other population-based study, from 2003, specifically focused on papillary kidney cancer (n = 1,733). It demonstrated a slightly wider range of SPCs with a significant excess risk – though the most dramatic result was still for bladder cancer (table 45) [4].

Augmenting these results, Thompson and colleagues noted in a 2006 report that patients with papillary renal cell carcinoma have an overall greater risk of a SPC, particularly related to colon and prostate cancer, than patients with clear cell renal carcinoma [5].

The theory concerning tobacco smoking and increased bladder cancer noted earlier may also explain any excess of second primary lung cancers. Consequently, smoking cessation could be an effective preventive measure. In the studies just described, prostate cancer joins the list of sites with excess risk, a result that has been confirmed by other research [3, 6]. No definitive explanation of this association has been offered.

Table 44. SPC following renal cell carcinoma

SPC	Overall SIR
NHL	2.47 (1.07–4.87)
Urinary bladder	2.09 (1.14–3.51)
Melanoma,skin	2.35 (1.13–4.33)
All cancers	**1.22 (1.03–1.45)**

Figures in parentheses are 95% CI. Adapted from Beisland et al. [1].

Table 45. SPC following renal papillary cancer by follow-up period

SPC	Overall SIR	Years of follow-up: SIR		
		<1 year	1–10 years	>10 years
Lung	2.47 (1.55–3.61)		2.21 (1.17–3.58)	
NHL	3.22 (1.28–6.05)		4.26 (1.53–8.35)	
Prostate	2.29 (1.71–2.96)	6.26 (3.11–10.51)	2.15 (1.46–2.98)	
Leukemia	2.80 (1.01–5.49)			
Urinary bladder	25.3 (21.5–29.5)	102.8 (76.8–132.7)	23.9 (19.3–28.9)	5.4 (2.5–9.5)
All cancers	**3.05 (2.73–3.40)**		**2.87 (2.49–3.29)**	**1.62 (1.18–2.13)**

Figures in parentheses are 95% CI. Adapted from Czene and Hemminki [4].

The most comprehensive study of this topic dates to 2002; it examined all types of kidney cancer (n = 23,137) [7]. As table 46 shows, the usual suspects already identified reappear as significant SPC risks. But the list is actually doubled in length, notably adding brain/central nervous system malignancy, leukemia as well as cancer of the endocrine glands and pancreas. Several of these new associations may be accounted for in terms of a familial syndrome involving a specific genetic defect [8].

Apart from bladder cancer, NHL is the only SPC with excess risk to appear in all 3 studies that we have detailed. A case series examined in 2006 added more evidence of an association between kidney cancer and NHL [9]. Despite this, the evidence of the association has certainly been debated, and the causal factors remain speculative [10, 11].

Bladder

The literature concerning SPC following bladder malignancies is even more modest than that seen with kidney cancer. Moreover, the topic frequently involves a

Table 46. SPC following cancer of the kidney

SPC	Overall SIR
Lung	1.36 (1.13–1.61)
Colon	1.39 (1.16–1.65)
Female breast	1.25 (1.04–1.48)
Pancreas	1.81 (1.40–2.27)
NHL	1.86 (1.42–2.36)
Brain/central nervous system	4.12 (3.38–4.93)
Prostate	1.70 (1.52–1.88)
Leukemia	2.45 (1.93–3.03)
Kidney	2.00 (1.57–2.49)
Urinary bladder	4.56 (4.04–5.12)
Endocrine glands	5.25 (4.18–6.44)
All cancers	**1.70 (1.63–1.78)**

Figures in parentheses are 95% CI. Adapted from Czene and Hemminki [7].

discussion of so-called transitional cell carcinoma of the upper urinary tract [12]. One study showed that the SIR for upper urinary tract tumors subsequent to bladder cancer was 51.3 (95% CI 47.5–55.4) [13]. As the risk factors for this association are not clear, targeted surveillance is the only recommended follow-up. The association is actually bidirectional, with an excess risk of bladder cancer following upper tract transitional cell carcinoma. This result will continue to prompt the search for a common risk factor [14].

An excess risk of prostate cancer appears to be the greatest concern in male bladder cancer survivors [15, 16]. A 2007 study indicated a SIR of 2.51 (95% CI 2.32–2.70), with the strongest impact in men diagnosed with first primary bladder cancer before age 60 [17]. In 2007, Italian research suggested an even higher SIR of 3.52 (95% CI 2.89–4.25) for second prostate cancer [18]. We should note that this association may also be bidirectional (but see the next section) [19].

An earlier study involving over 10,000 bladder cancer patients derived a SIR of 1.31 (95% CI 1.13–1.50) for subsequent lung cancer and 3.55 (95% CI 1.84–6.20) for kidney cancer in women. These risks, which persisted for 20 years, were partly related to smoking [20]. Adding to the data, a recent German study (n = 1,260) indicated an excess risk for prostate and lung cancer (in men) and breast and colon cancer (in women) following bladder cancer [21]. Finally, the 2007 Italian study cited above also suggested excess second kidney tumors in male bladder cancer survivors (significant SIR = 3.90) [18]. At the least, long-term surveillance is strongly recommended.

Table 47. SPC and synchronous cancer following prostate cancer

SPC	Overall SIR
Colon	1.24 (1.17–1.31)
Pancreas	1.15 (1.05–1.26)
Brain	1.62 (1.44–1.81)
Leukemia/lymphoma	1.13 (1.05–1.20)
Kidney	1.52 (1.40–1.65)
Urinary bladder	1.59 (1.51–1.68)
Melanoma	1.33 (1.17–1.50)
Liver	1.20 (1.09–1.32)
Small intestine	2.20 (1.83–2.61)
Male breast	2.01 (1.44–2.74)
Endocrine gland	1.81 (1.51–2.16)

Figures in parentheses are 95% CI. Adapted from Thellenberg et al. [24].

Prostate

As early as 1985, researchers had concluded that 'in contrast to other index tumors, the prostate stands out as being associated with an overall low risk of second cancer development' [22]. Indeed, confirming other research, a 1999 study actually reported a deficiency of SPC following prostate cancer [23]. Such results may be erroneous, resulting from biases such as reduced surveillance in elderly men with prostate carcinoma.

Nonetheless, a large study (n = 135,713) in 2003 concluded that observed SPCs were less than expected, though this specifically applied when incident cases in the first 6 months of follow-up were removed (that is, eliminating synchronous tumors, according to a stricter cutoff than the 2-month standard we are following). One rationale for not including the first 6 months of cases in any SPC research, apart from basic definitional considerations, is that it tends to lessen the impact of surveillance bias. On the other hand, the conservative 6-month cutoff runs the risk of missing true SPC cases and thus not recognizing legitimate risk associations.

If the first 6 months of follow-up are included in this study (that is, the data presumably incorporate synchronous cancers, by any definition), then a number of cancers show a statistically significant increase, as indicated in table 47 [24].

This study demonstrates that the statistical effect of eliminating synchronous tumors can be substantial. If only metachronous tumors are considered (according to the researchers' definition those cancers arising after 6 months), the list of SPCs of significant excess is substantially reduced (table 48). Cancer of the male breast is the standout example of second primary malignancy. Considering etiology, breast and

Table 48. SPC following prostate cancer

SPC	Overall SIR
Melanoma	1.33 (1.16–1.51)
Small intestine	1.39 (1.09–1.75)
Male breast	1.95 (1.36–2.71)
Endocrine gland	1.41 (1.13–1.74)

Figures in parentheses are 95% CI. Adapted from Thellenberg et al. [24].

prostate cancer may be associated either by genetic or treatment effects, the latter specifically referring to estrogen therapy used in the treatment of prostate cancer.

There has been mixed evidence of increased bladder cancer following prostate cancer [25]. A review in 2004 found that only 3 of 11 studies supported the conclusion that an excess risk exists [19]. However, a small 2005 study did add to the data indicating an association. It calculated a SIR of 4.31 (95% CI 2.41–7.11) [26]. Likewise, a 2007 study that combined data from 5 cancer registries suggested that there was an increased rate of bladder cancer, but only in men younger than 60 years [17]. Finally, another 2007 study linked an increased risk of bladder cancer specifically to smoking (with an additional synergistic effect in the face of radiation for prostate cancer) [27].

A well-studied subtopic in this area has focused on whether or not full-dose radiotherapy for prostate cancer induces SPC in adjacent tissues. A study based on over 51,000 men suggested a small but significantly increased risk of solid tumors when comparing radiotherapy against surgery [28].

On another front, a study based on the British Columbia Tumour Registry looked at 29,371 prostate cancer patients who did not receive radiotherapy and 9,890 who did receive radiation. Certain solid tumors were found in significant excess in the radiotherapy group; this result also held when compared against the nonradiotherapy cohort, specifically for colorectal cancer and pelvic bone and connective tissue sarcoma. Cancer of the testis and bladder was also elevated significantly over normal expectations, but only in the nonradiotherapy group [29].

These findings should be compared against the wider literature, which has consistently indicated zero to (at most) modest excess risks of SPC following irradiation [30]. Consistent with the general SPC results noted earlier, bladder cancer in particular does not seem to be significantly and substantially elevated following radiation for prostate cancer [31, 32]. Finally, adding to this complex narrative, a recent study showed a SIR of 1.7 (95% CI 1.4–2.2) for rectal cancer in 30,552 patients who underwent radiotherapy for prostate cancer, whereas a 2006 analysis of an even larger pool of patients did not demonstrate any such increased risk [33, 34].

Table 49. SPC following testicular cancer

SPC	Overall SIR [43]
Lung	1.5 (1.2–1.7)
Colon	2.0 (1.7–2.5)
Rectum	1.8 (1.4–2.3)
Pancreas	3.6 (2.8–4.6)
Prostate	1.4 (1.2–1.6)
Stomach	4.0 (3.2–4.8)
Kidney	2.4 (1.8–3.0)
Urinary bladder	2.7 (2.2–3.1)
Melanoma, skin	1.8 (1.3–2.3)
Connective tissue	4.0 (2.3–6.3)
Pleura	3.4 (1.7–5.9)
Other solid tumors	1.6 (1.4–1.9)
All solid tumors	**1.9 (1.8–2.1)**

Figures in parentheses are 95% CI. Adapted from Travis et al. [42].

In sum, little has changed the reality of the 1999 assessment by Levi et al. [23] that the public health impact of SPC following prostate cancer is at most modest. This general assessment does not appreciably change when studies isolate the effect of radiotherapy [35]. Whatever SPC risks are attributable to radiation, recent research has indicated that the impact may be ameliorated by newer therapeutic techniques, such as the use of radioactive implants [36, 37].

Testis

The data for second cancers following testicular cancer have been clear and consistent compared to the other parts of the male genitourinary tract. Most testicular cancers are germ cell tumors of 2 main histological types, seminomas and teratomas. Of the 2, seminomas are most often implicated in the SPC story [38].

The phenomenon of excess cancers following treatment for testicular cancer has been well known for 10 years [39]. The best established associations are radiotherapy (connected with second solid tumors in the radiation field) and chemotherapy (linked with second leukemias) [40]. However, given that testicular cancer is the most common solid tumor among young males (aged 15–35 years), the high cure rates continue to suggest that treatment benefits vastly outweigh the increased risk of SPC [41]. This assessment even applies to intense treatments such as the high-dose chemotherapy applied before stem cell transplantation.

Table 50. SPC following testicular cancer

SPC	Overall SIR		
	all histologies	seminomas	nonseminomas
Lung	1.33 (1.17–1.52)	1.35 (1.17–1.56)	
Colorectal	1.45 (1.26–1.67)	1.54 (1.31–1.79)	
Colon	1.51 (1.25–1.82)	1.54 (1.24–1.89)	
Rectum	1.37 (1.09–1.71)	1.53 (1.19–1.93)	
Pancreas	2.56 (2.03–3.19)	2.45 (1.87–3.15)	2.98 (1.79–4.65)
NHL	1.65 (1.27–2.10)	1.79 (1.33–2.36)	
Leukemia			
Myeloid leukemia	3.62 (2.56–4.97)	2.39 (1.41–3.77)	6.77 (4.14–10.50)
Other leukemia	3.47 (2.20–5.21)	3.48 (2.03–5.57)	3.44 (1.26–7.48)
Esophagus	1.79 (1.20–2.57)	1.90 (1.22–2.82)	
Stomach	2.37 (1.97–2.82)	2.25 (1.82–2.75)	2.85 (1.92–4.07)
Kidney	2.05 (1.62–2.56)	2.02 (1.53–2.60)	2.17 (1.30–3.38)
Bladder	2.12 (1.80–2.47)	2.27 (1.91–2.68)	
Thyroid	2.86 (1.69–4.51)	3.06 (1.63–5.23)	
Gallbladder	2.01 (1.10–3.37)	2.17 (1.12–3.79)	
Melanoma, skin	1.62 (1.29–2.01)	1.77 (1.35–2.27)	
Soft tissue sarcoma	2.63 (1.58–4.11)		4.00 (1.83–7.60)
Nonmelanoma skin	2.26 (1.97–2.57)	2.17 (1.85–2.53)	2.54 (1.94–3.27)
All cancers	**1.65 (1.57–1.73)**	**1.63 (1.55–1.72)**	**1.71 (1.55–1.88)**

Figures in parentheses are 95% CI. Adapted from Richiardi et al. [49].

In 2005, Travis and colleagues updated their research from the 1990s. They examined 40,476 testicular cancer survivors, generating the evidence of excess solid tumors shown in table 49 [42].

The analysis further indicated that the risk remained elevated at some sites for decades. A 2007 study in the Netherlands confirmed that prolonged follow-up was required after both radiotherapy and chemotherapy for testicular cancer, possibly for as long as 20 years [44].

A 2001 report from the research group associated with the Swedish Family Cancer Database strongly confirmed the results provided above for pancreatic and bladder tumors following testicular cancer. The former is particularly serious from a prognostic perspective. The SIR for all SPCs in this study was 1.6 (95% CI 1.4–1.9) [38].

Augmenting the results just described, another study group led by Travis reported an excess of leukemia following both chemotherapy and radiotherapy for testicular cancer [45]. Based on what was once the standard radiation regimen, the estimated SIR was 3.2 (95% CI 1.5–8.4). Overall, the cumulative incidence of leukemia remains moderate, but even the relatively low number of SPCs should not prevent 'the search for equally effective but less toxic therapies' [46]. In fact, treatment improvements have been achieved in recent years [47, 48].

Many of the key results obtained in the research by Travis and coauthors were confirmed by a 2007 British study that examined 5,555 seminoma patients and 3,733 nonseminoma patients [47]. Pancreatic cancer was a standout among both cohorts, especially over the long-term (SIR = 5.48 for seminomas; SIR = 10.17 for nonseminomatous testicular cancer). Notably, leukemia was found in significant excess over the short-term following both types of testicular cancer.

The most recent larger analysis of SPC following testicular cancer was completed in 2006. The results generated in the investigation of 29,511 patients from 13 cancer registries confirmed many of the excess risks described above and added several others (table 50) [49].

The record of a remarkably consistent excess risk seen for malignancies following testicular cancer is maintained in this latest research. Richiardi and colleagues point out that most studies have pegged the SIR for all SPC between 1.20 and 1.60. This fact positions testicular cancer as one of the key candidates for new therapies with more benign late effects or, failing that, intensive long-term surveillance.

Notes and References

1 Beisland C, Talleraas O, Bakke A, et al: Multiple primary malignancies in patients with renal cell carcinoma: a national population-based cohort study. BJU Int 2006;97:698–702.

2 Rabbani F, Grimaldi G, Russo P: Multiple primary malignancies in renal cell carcinoma. J Urol 1998; 160:1255–1259.

3 McCredie M, Macfarlane GJ, Stewart J, et al: Second primary cancers following cancers of the kidney and prostate in New South Wales (Australia), 1972–91. Cancer Causes Control 1996;7:337–344.

4 Czene K, Hemminki K: Familial papillary renal cell tumors and subsequent cancers: a nationwide epidemiological study from Sweden. J Urol 2003;169: 1271–1275.

5 Thompson RH, Leibovich BC, Cheville JC, et al: Second primary malignancies associated with renal cell carcinoma histological subtypes. J Urol 2006;176: 900–903; discussion 903–904.

6 Barocas DA, Rabbani F, Scherr DS, et al: A population-based study of renal cell carcinoma and prostate cancer in the same patients. BJU Int 2006;97: 33–36.

7 Czene K, Hemminki K: Kidney cancer in the Swedish Family Cancer Database: familial risks and second primary malignancies. Kidney Int 2002;61:1806–1813.

8 Wagner JR, Linehan WM: Molecular genetics of renal cell carcinoma. Semin Urol Oncol 1996;14: 244–249.

9 Kunthur A, Wiernik PH, Dutcher JP: Renal parenchymal tumors and lymphoma in the same patient: case series and review of the literature. Am J Hematol 2006;81:271–280.

10 Rabbani F, Russo P: Lack of association between renal cell carcinoma and non-Hodgkin's lymphoma. Urology 1999;54:28–33.

11 Anderson CM, Pusztai L, Palmer JL, et al: Coincident renal cell carcinoma and non-Hodgkin's lymphoma: the M.D. Anderson experience and review of the literature. J Urol 1998;159:714–717.
12 Defined as the tissue in the kidneys that collects urine (the renal pelvis) and the ureters.
13 Rabbani F, Perrotti M, Russo P, et al: Upper-tract tumors after an initial diagnosis of bladder cancer: argument for long-term surveillance. J Clin Oncol 2001;19:94–100.
14 Raman JD, Ng CK, Boorjian SA, et al: Bladder cancer after managing upper urinary tract transitional cell carcinoma: predictive factors and pathology. BJU Int 2005;96:1031–1035.
15 Kurokawa K, Ito K, Yamamoto T, et al: Comparative study on the prevalence of clinically detectable prostate cancer in patients with and without bladder cancer. Urology 2004;63:268–272.
16 Kotake T, Kiyohara H: Multiple primary cancers (MPC) associated with bladder cancer: an analysis of the clinical and autopsy cases in Japan. Jpn J Clin Oncol 1985;15(suppl 1):201–210.
17 Kellen E, Zeegers MP, Dirx M, et al: Occurrence of both bladder and prostate cancer in five cancer registries in Belgium, the Netherlands and the United Kingdom. Eur J Cancer 2007;43:1694–1700.
18 Fabbri C, Ravaioli A, Ravaioli A, et al: Risk of cancer of the prostate and of the kidney parenchyma following bladder cancer. Tumori 2007;93:124–128.
19 Kinoshita Y, Singh A, Rovito PM Jr, et al: Double primary cancers of the prostate and bladder: a literature review. Clin Prost Cancer 2004;3:83–86.
20 Salminen E, Pukkala E, Teppo L: Bladder cancer and the risk of smoking-related cancers during followup. J Urol 1994;152:1420–1423.
21 Klotz T, Hofstadter F, Gerken M: Interdisciplinary oncologic after-care exemplified by second primary tumors after bladder carcinoma. Urologe A 2003;42: 1485–1490.
22 Kleinerman RA, Liebermann JV, Li FP: Second cancer following cancer of the male genital system in Connecticut, 1935–82. Natl Cancer Inst Monogr 1985;68:139–147.
23 Levi F, Randimbison L, Te V, et al: Second primary tumors after prostate carcinoma. Cancer 1999;86: 1567–1570.
24 Thellenberg C, Malmer B, Tavelin B, et al: Second primary cancers in men with prostate cancer: an increased risk of male breast cancer. J Urol 2003;169:1345–1348.
25 Goldstraw MA, Payne H, Kirby RS: What are the risks of second cancer formation after radiotherapy to the prostate? BJU Int 2006;98:489–491.
26 Singh A, Kinoshita Y, Rovito PM Jr, et al: Higher than expected association of clinical prostate and bladder cancers. J Urol 2005;173:1526–1529.
27 Boorjian S, Cowan JE, Konety BR, et al: Bladder cancer incidence and risk factors in men with prostate cancer: results from Cancer of the Prostate Strategic Urologic Research Endeavor. J Urol 2007;177:883–887; discussion 887–888.
28 Brenner DJ, Curtis RE, Hall EJ, et al: Second malignancies in prostate carcinoma patients after radiotherapy compared with surgery. Cancer 2000;88: 398–406.
29 Pickles T, Phillips N: The risk of second malignancy in men with prostate cancer treated with or without radiation in British Columbia, 1984–2000. Radiother Oncol 2002;65:145–151.
30 Movsas B, Hanlon AL, Pinover W, et al: Is there an increased risk of second primaries following prostate irradiation? Int J Radiat Oncol Biol Phys 1998;41: 251–255.
31 Neugut AI, Ahsan H, Robinson E: Bladder carcinoma and other second malignancies after radiotherapy for prostate carcinoma. Cancer 1997:79: 1600–1604.
32 Chrouser K, Leibovich B, Bergstralh E, et al: Bladder cancer risk following primary and adjuvant external beam radiation for prostate cancer. J Urol 2005;174:107–110; discussion 110–111.
33 Baxter NN, Tepper JE, Durham SB, et al: Increased risk of rectal cancer after prostate radiation: a population-based study. Gastroenterology 2005;128: 819–824.
34 Kendal WS, Eapen L, Macrae R, et al: Prostatic irradiation is not associated with any measurable increase in the risk of subsequent rectal cancer. Int J Radiat Oncol Biol Phys 2006;65:661–668.
35 Liauw SL, Sylvester JE, Morris CG, et al: Second malignancies after prostate brachytherapy: incidence of bladder and colorectal cancers in patients with 15 years of potential follow-up. Int J Radiat Oncol Biol Phys 2006;66:669–673.
36 Moon K, Stukenborg GJ, Keim J, et al: Cancer incidence after localized therapy for prostate cancer. Cancer 2006;107:991–998.
37 Schneider U, Lomax A, Besserer J, et al: The impact of dose escalation on secondary cancer risk after radiotherapy of prostate cancer. Int J Radiat Oncol Biol Phys 2007;68:892–897.
38 Dong C, Lonnstedt I, Hemminki K: Familial testicular cancer and second primary cancers in testicular cancer patients by histological type. Eur J Cancer 2001;37:1878–1885.
39 Nichols CR, Loehrer PJ Sr: The story of second cancers in patients cured of testicular cancer: tarnishing success or burnishing irrelevance? J Natl Cancer Inst 1997;89:1394–1395.
40 Fossa SD: Long-term sequelae after cancer therapy – survivorship after treatment for testicular cancer. Acta Oncol 2004;43:134–141.

41 Chaudhary UB, Haldas JR: Long-term complications of chemotherapy for germ cell tumours. Drugs 2003;63:1565–1577.
42 Travis LB, Fossa SD, Schonfeld SJ, et al: Second cancers among 40,576 testicular cancer patients: focus on long-term survivors. J Natl Cancer Inst 2005;97:1354–1365.
43 After at least 10 years of follow-up.
44 Van den Belt-Dusebout AW, de Wit R, Gietema JA, et al: Treatment-specific risks of second malignancies and cardiovascular disease in 5-year survivors of testicular cancer. J Clin Oncol 2007;25:4370–4378.
45 Travis LB, Andersson M, Gospodarowicz M, et al: Treatment-associated leukemia following testicular cancer. J Natl Cancer Inst 2000;92:1165–1171.
46 Kollmannsberger C, Hartmann JT, Kanz L, et al: Therapy-related malignancies following treatment of germ cell cancer. Int J Cancer 1999;83:860–863.
47 Robinson D, Moller H, Horwich A: Mortality and incidence of second cancers following treatment for testicular cancer. Br J Cancer 2007;96:529–533.
48 Schairer C, Hisada M, Chen BE, et al: Comparative mortality for 621 second cancers in 29,356 testicular cancer survivors and 12,420 matched first cancers. J Natl Cancer Inst 2007;99:1248–1256.
49 Richiardi L, Scelo G, Boffetta P, et al: Second malignancies among survivors of germ-cell testicular cancer: a pooled analysis between 13 cancer registries. Int J Cancer 2007;120:623–631.

Krueger H, McLean D, Williams D: The Prevention of Second Primary Cancers.
Prog Exp Tumor Res. Basel, Karger, 2008, vol 40, pp 102–110

12

Gynecologic Cancers

Within gynecologic oncology, the best data for SPC risks are available for ovarian and cervical cancer, though some information is available for uterine (endometrial) and vulvar malignancies as well. An extension in this area was provided in 2007 with the first substantial research on SPC following fallopian tube cancer.

Ovary

A research team led by Hemminki studied Swedish registry data for 19,440 ovarian carcinomas. Table 51 shows a significant excess for all SPC, with the most notable results for specific malignancies seen with colorectal, pancreatic, stomach, kidney and bladder cancer, as well as leukemia [1].

Contrary to the nonsignificant results for second breast cancer, other, earlier studies have demonstrated a significant SIR for breast tumors following ovarian cancer [2]. However, a 2007 study of 45,986 cases of epithelial ovarian cancer (plus 3,297 cases of a rare form of neoplasm known as low malignant potential tumor) drawn from the SEER database drew a different conclusion, actually suggesting a protective effect on second breast cancer (SIR = 0.72, 95% CI 0.52–0.98) [3]. The main explanation for such an effect is the medical or surgical therapy for ovarian cancer offering a concomitant benefit in terms of reduced breast cancer development.

Many of the excess SPCs are attributed to therapy effects in the other direction, even though this does not always appear to be borne out by the SIR trends over long-term follow-up observed in this study. Hereditary nonpolyposis colorectal cancer syndrome, described earlier in the context of gastrointestinal first primaries, may play a role in the excess intestinal, stomach, kidney and bladder cancers found following ovarian tumors (and endometrial tumors, see below).

The options for prevention of SPC appear to be limited, mostly related to making therapy as safe as possible. As usual, targeted surveillance is indicated following treatment for a first primary. On the specific topic of breast cancer following ovarian carcinoma, one researcher concluded that, in patients without a genetic predisposition,

Table 51. SPC following ovarian carcinoma by follow-up period

SPC	Overall SIR	Years of follow-up: SIR		
		<1 year	1–10 years	>10 years
Colon	1.90 (1.59–2.24)	5.52		1.93
Rectum	1.97 (1.53–2.51)		1.91	2.26
Breast	1.10 (0.97–1.25) (NS)			
Pancreas	1.75 (1.29–2.32)		1.67	1.72
Leukemia	2.27 (1.68–3.02)		3.05	
Stomach	1.60 (1.16–2.16)	3.24		1.76
Kidney	1.77 (1.29–2.38)	7.22		
Urinary bladder	1.99 (1.43–2.69)			2.19
Uterus	1.76 (1.43–2.15)	12.74	0.63	
Thyroid gland	1.78 (1.02–2.90)			
Connective tissue	3.40 (2.01–5.39)		3.47	3.48
Small intestine	3.08 (1.59–5.41)	13.79	2.90	
Nonmelanoma skin cancer	1.61 (1.15–2.20)			
All cancers	**1.47 (1.39–1.56)**	**2.95**	**1.28**	**1.45**

Figures in parentheses are 95% CI. NS = Not significant. Adapted from Hemminki et al. [1].

'additional mammography examinations based on the assumption of an increased risk of breast cancer are not warranted in ovarian cancer patients' [4].

The most recent comprehensive examination of MPCs following ovarian cancer demonstrated a similar range of cases to that shown by Hemminki and colleagues. However, the SIRs were much higher, probably because the topic was concurrent tumors, that is, those developing within 1 year of the first primary [5]. This means that metastases would be included in the results. Despite the different focus, additional weight was added to the search for common etiologies and biomarkers between ovarian and endometrial cancers, in particular.

Fallopian Tube

Primary fallopian tube cancer is a rare disease, possibly explaining why SPC has not been a serious topic of investigation. In 2007, Riska and colleagues examined 2,084 cases of fallopian tube cancer drawn from 13 cancer registries from Europe, Australia, Canada and Singapore [6]. They demonstrated very modest excess risks of SPC overall and a few specific cancers (table 52). The main etiologic linkages suggested are smoking (related to bladder cancer) and genetic risk factors (related to colorectal and breast cancers).

Table 52. SPC following fallopian tube cancer

SPC	Overall SIR
Colorectal	1.7 (1.0–2.6)
Breast	1.5 (1.1–2.2)
Leukemia	
Nonlymphoid	3.7 (1.0–9.4)
Bladder	2.8 (1.0–6.0)
All cancers	**1.4 (1.1–1.6)**

Figures in parentheses are 95% CI. Adapted from Riska et al. [6].

Table 53. SPC following endometrial carcinoma by follow-up period

SPC	Overall SIR	Years of follow-up: SIR		
		<1 year	1–10 years	>10 years
Colon	1.84 (1.64–2.07)	2.87	1.57	2.07
Rectum	1.99 (1.68–2.35)	2.99	1.68	2.27
Breast	1.39 (1.28–1.51)	2.56	1.40	1.22
Ovary	3.16 (2.80–3.56)	55.77	0.67	0.22
Leukemia	1.37 (1.04–1.76)		1.48	
Kidney	1.65 (1.32–2.05)	3.57	1.42	1.76
Urinary bladder	2.35 (1.92–2.84)		1.90	2.88
Other female genitals	1.99 (1.37–2.80)			2.70
Connective tissue	2.03 (1.25–3.11)		2.15	
Small intestine	2.00 (1.14–3.25)	14.71		
Nonmelanoma skin cancer	1.54 (1.23–1.90)		1.61	1.51
All cancers	**1.54 (1.48–1.61)**	**5.59**	**1.30**	**1.43**

Figures in parentheses are 95% CI. Adapted from Hemminki et al. [1].

Endometrium

Both radiotherapy and chemotherapy are used more with ovarian than endometrial cancer, which may account for the smaller SIRs related to connective tissue malignancies and leukemia following endometrial cancer (table 53) [1].

The data show that breast cancer was significantly elevated after endometrial cancer, differing from the result seen for ovarian cancer in the same 2003 study by Hemminki

Table 54. SPC following in situ vulvar cancer

SPC	Overall SIR
Lung	3.2
Pharynx	5.0
Larynx	8.0
Anus	17.3
Endocrine glands	17.9
All cancers	**1.5**

Adapted from Sturgeon et al. [8].

Table 55. SPC following invasive vulvar cancer

SPC	Overall SIR
Lung	2.1
NHL	2.1
Brain/central nervous system	3.1
Melanoma, skin	2.8
Anus	6.0
All cancers	**1.3**

Adapted from Sturgeon et al. [8].

and colleagues. Hormonal factors are posited as an explanation for this difference. Hormones have also been suggested as the mechanism behind the bidirectional association observed between ovarian and endometrial carcinomas. Risk factors that perhaps should intensify surveillance efforts in endometrial cancer patients include menopause occurring after age 51 and obesity [7].

Vulva and Vagina

The data for SPC following vulvar and vaginal cancer do not seem to have been updated for 10 years. There are basically no significant SIR results related to vaginal malignancy, but Sturgeon et al. [8] did derive relevant information for first primary vulvar cancer (both in situ and invasive types). This study did not supply the 95% CI, but did identify the significant values ($p < 0.05$). The results are provided in tables 54 and 55.

The 2 most important risk factors involved with SPC following vulvar cancer are thought to be tobacco use (leading to lung and pharyngeal cancers, among others) and infection with HPV (accounting for the excess risk of anal cancer, for instance).

Table 56. SPC following invasive cervical cancer

SPC	Overall SIR
Lung	3.1
Breast	0.8
Stomach	1.8
Pharynx	2.0
Urinary bladder	2.4
Melanoma, skin	0.5
Uterus	0.5
Larynx	2.4
Anus	4.7
Vulva	5.2
Vagina	13.6
Bone	5.7
All cancers	**1.3**

Adapted from Sturgeon et al. [8].

Control of 1 or both of these factors would presumably reduce the risk of SPC following vulvar and other lower genital tract cancers [9].

Cervical Cancer

The early study by Sturgeon and coauthors on vulvar cancer cited in the previous section indicated that identical etiologic relationships are at work in cervical cancer, demonstrated by the substantial excess of SPCs detected in the lung, anus, vulva and vagina (table 56).

The protective effect suggested here for second breast cancer has been confirmed in other, though not all, studies [10]. A very large analysis from 2007 supported the idea of a protective effect (table 61). The key explanations revolve around variations in hormonal exposure experienced by breast tissues as a result of factors related to pregnancy history and therapy in cervical cancer patients [11].

Two different European studies from the early 2000s continued the cervical cancer SPC story. Both papers included information for invasive cervical cancer and its precursor conditions. The data derived by Hemminki and colleagues for 117,830 Swedish subjects with in situ cancer follow the now familiar pattern, with SPCs largely focused on sites susceptible to tobacco exposure and HPV infection (table 57) [12].

If anything, the study by Evans et al. [13] found an even closer match with the expected pattern among 59,519 cases of cervical intraepithelial neoplasia III. Table 58

Table 57. SPC following in situ cervical cancer

SPC	Overall SIR
Upper aerodigestive tract	1.57 (1.28–1.89)
Lung	2.17 (2.00–2.34)
Pancreas	1.22 (1.02–1.43)
Leukemia	1.27 (1.08–1.48)
Esophagus	1.85 (1.25–2.57)
Stomach	1.22 (1.03–1.43)
Urinary bladder	1.39 (1.17–1.63)
Anus	3.75 (2.91–4.69)
Other female genitals	3.68 (3.12–4.28)
Nonmelanoma skin cancer	1.26 (1.04–1.50)
All cancers	**1.17 (1.15–1.20)**

Figures in parentheses are 95% CI. Adapted from Hemminki et al. [12].

Table 58. SPC following cervical intraepithelial neoplasia III

SPC	Overall SIR
Lung	1.8 (1.5–2.1)
Anus	5.9 (3.7–8.8)
Vulva	4.4 (2.8–6.6)
Vagina	18.5 (13.0–25.5)
All cancers	**1.2 (1.2–1.3)**

Figures in parentheses are 95% CI. Adapted from Evans et al. [13].

shows the excess SPCs coordinated exactly with the etiologic factors we have been discussing, that is, tobacco smoking and HPV infection.

The results from both studies for invasive forms of cervical cancer only reinforce the common role of tobacco use and HPV infection in driving excess SPC incidence. Hemminki and colleagues based their results on 17,556 cases (table 59); table 60 shows the analysis by Evans and colleagues of a somewhat larger sample (n = 21,605).

The ongoing, intense interest in all matters concerning cervical cancer continues to be extended to SPC research. About half a dozen major studies were published on this specific topic in 2007. For instance, data on 104,760 survivors of cervical cancer drawn from 13 population-based registries generated the following significant SIR information (table 61) [11].

It is important to note that all tables in this section have confirmed the same relatively modest SIR for all SPC, namely, 1.2–1.3. In this respect, the most serious prevention and surveillance efforts perhaps should be focused on the sites where the SIRs are most substantial, notably in the anogenital region. A 2007 Swedish study confirmed that cancers of the vagina, vulva and anus are a particular concern following a diagnosis of cervical intraepithelial neoplasia [14]. It is convenient to introduce at this point the fact that anal cancer as a first primary has generated a small body of literature, suggesting a pattern of bidirectional SPC risks. Excess incidence of tumors following anal cancer has been observed in the lung and vulva/vagina, among other sites [15]. Again, common environmental risk factors such as smoking and/or viral infection seem to be the likely etiologic explanation. Given the growing understanding

Table 59. SPC following invasive cervical cancer

SPC	Overall SIR
Upper aerodigestive tract	1.85 (1.27–2.53)
Lung	2.81 (2.43–3.21)
Colon	1.30 (1.10–1.51)
Rectum	1.91 (1.57–2.28)
Breast	0.77 (0.68–0.85)
Pancreas	1.35 (1.03–1.70)
Urinary bladder	4.15 (3.51–4.84)
Liver	0.66 (0.46–0.90)
Anus	3.92 (2.28–6.00)
Other female genitals	4.80 (3.72–6.02)
Connective tissue	2.27 (1.44–3.30)
All cancers	**1.25 (1.19–1.30)**

Figures in parentheses are 95% CI. Adapted from Hemminki et al. [12].

Table 60. SPC following invasive cervical cancer

SPC	Overall SIR
Lung	2.5 (2.2–2.8)
Rectum	1.4 (1.1–1.9)
Urinary bladder	1.7 (1.3–2.3)
Anus	6.3 (3.7–10.0)
Vulva	1.9 (1.0–3.3)
Vagina	8.0 (4.4–13.5)
Connective tissue	2.7 (1.2–5.3)
All cancers	**1.2 (1.1–1.2)**

Figures in parentheses are 95% CI. Adapted from: Evans et al. [13].

of HPV infection and carcinogenesis in the head and neck region, it is not surprising that elevated risks of cancer in the oropharynx and larynx following cervical cancer were confirmed in a smaller SEER analysis published in 2008 [16].

In addition to the standard call for caution around smoking and the sexual transmission of HPV, there is also a therapy dimension to the follow-up of first primary cervical cancer. Radiation is a common form of treatment for invasive cervical cancer, and the evidence has been accumulating for 20 years of excess cancer risk in irradiated sites. In a 1995 study, a therapy effect was observed for rectal, vaginal, vulvar, ovarian and bladder cancers. Additionally, excess risk was evident for kidney and bone cancer as well as leukemia [17]. The result for leukemia was also reflected in the study by Hemminki and colleagues of in situ cervical cancer described earlier. Furthermore, the large 2007 study introduced above strongly confirmed the impact of radiation on sites near the cervix, specifically external genitals, the bladder and the rectum. The apparent overall protective effect of a first primary cervical cancer on tumors of the uterine corpus and the ovary appears to yield to a negative impact of therapy at later years of follow-up [11].

Given the proven effectiveness as measured by survival, recent Japanese studies of radiotherapy for cervical cancer concluded that the benefits of current interventions already outweigh any risks related to SPC and other complications [18, 19]. However, in light of the apparent late effects of treatment, a 2006 report offered the hope that 'analyses of genetic susceptibility and molecular carcinogenesis can be used to develop more

Table 61. SPC following cervical cancer by follow-up period

SPC	Overall SIR	Years of follow-up: SIR				
		1–9 years	10–19 years	20–29 years	30–39 years	≥40 years
Lung	2.57 (2.47–2.70)	4.23	2.34	1.73	1.54	0.80
Colorectal						
Colon	1.22 (1.16–1.30)	1.25		1.23		1.67
Rectum/anus	1.84 (1.72–1.98)		2.01	2.23	3.09	5.79
Female breast	0.77 (0.74–0.81)	0.78	0.70	0.60	0.59	0.90
Pancreas	1.37 (1.25–1.50)	1.63			1.47	
NHL	1.27 (1.14–1.42)					
Ovary	0.88 (0.81–0.97)	0.61	0.98	1.22	1.73	2.72
Leukemia						
Acute nonlymphocytic	1.72 (1.43–2.06)	2.74				
Esophagus	1.42 (1.16–1.73)					
Stomach	1.30 (1.19–1.43)	1.32	1.34	1.30		
Kidney	1.35 (1.22–1.51)			1.72	1.69	
Oral	1.48 (1.15–1.89)					
Pharynx	1.83 (1.37–2.41)					
Bladder	3.44 (3.23–3.67)	2.70	2.84	4.13	5.44	5.83
Melanoma, skin	0.74 (0.65–0.86)					
Larynx	2.02 (1.53–2.63)					
Uterus	0.74 (0.68–0.81)	0.48		1.27		
Other female genitals	4.81 (4.40–5.25)	4.00	4.01	5.54	6.33	8.66
Small intestine	1.80 (1.39–2.31)					
Soft tissue	2.53 (2.10–3.05)	2.41	3.63	2.24	4.05	
Bone	2.70 (1.85–3.82)	2.86	3.63			
Lip	1.66 (1.13–2.36)					
All cancers	**1.30 (1.28–1.33)**	**1.31**	**1.27**	**1.37**	**1.50**	**1.83**

Figures in parentheses are 95% CI. Adapted from Chaturvedi et al. [11].

appropriate strategies for radiation therapy for cervical cancers' [20]. In the meantime, one of the important results of the 2007 multiregistry analysis that we have been regularly citing is the demonstration that effects attributed to therapy are detectable beyond the 40-year point, thus indicating the need for surveillance over many decades [11].

Notes and References

1 Hemminki K, Aaltonen L, Li X: Subsequent primary malignancies after endometrial carcinoma and ovarian carcinoma. Cancer 2003;97:2432–2439.
2 For example, see Travis LB, Curtis RE, Boice JD Jr, et al: Second malignant neoplasms among long-term survivors of ovarian cancer. Cancer Res 1996;56: 1564–1570.
3 Hunter MI, Ziogas A, Flores F, et al: Epithelial ovarian cancer and low malignant potential (LMP) tumors associated with a lower incidence of second primary breast cancer. Am J Clin Oncol 2007;30: 1–7.
4 Bergfeldt K, Nilsson B, Einhorn S, et al: Breast cancer risk in women with a primary ovarian cancer–a case-control study. Eur J Cancer 2001;37:2229–2234.
5 Van Niekerk CC, Vooijs GP, Bulten J, et al: Increased risk of concurrent primary malignancies in patients diagnosed with a primary malignant epithelial ovarian tumor. Mod Pathol 2007;20:384–388.
6 Riska A, Pukkala E, Scelo G, et al: Second primary malignancies in females with primary fallopian tube cancer. Int J Cancer 2007;120:2047–2051.
7 Studzinski Z, Branicka D: The coexistence of endometrial cancer with second primary malignant neoplasms. Ginekol Pol 1999;70:186–192.
8 Sturgeon SR, Curtis RE, Johnson K, et al: Second primary cancers after vulvar and vaginal cancers. Am J Obstet Gynecol 1996;174:929–933.
9 Levi F, Randimbison L, La Vecchia C: Descriptive epidemiology of vulvar and vaginal cancers in Vaud, Switzerland, 1974–1994. Ann Oncol 1998;9: 1229–1232.
10 Werner-Wasik M, Schmid CH, Bornstein LE, et al: Increased risk of second malignant neoplasms outside radiation fields in patients with cervical carcinoma. Cancer 1995;75:2281–2285.
11 Chaturvedi AK, Engels EA, Gilbert ES, et al: Second cancers among 104,760 survivors of cervical cancer: evaluation of long-term risk. J Natl Cancer Inst 2007;99:1634–1643.
12 Hemminki K, Dong C, Vaittinen P: Second primary cancer after in situ and invasive cervical cancer. Epidemiology 2000;11:457–461.
13 Evans HS, Newnham A, Hodgson SV, et al: Second primary cancers after cervical intraepithelial neoplasia III and invasive cervical cancer in Southeast England. Gynecol Oncol 2003;90:131–136.
14 Edgren G, Sparen P: Risk of anogenital cancer after diagnosis of cervical intraepithelial neoplasia: a prospective population-based study. Lancet Oncol 2007;8:311–316.
15 Frisch M, Olsen JH, Melbye M: Malignancies before and after anal cancer: clues to their etiology. Am J Epidemiol 1994;140:12–19.
16 Rose Ragin CC, Taioli E: Second primary head and neck tumor risk in patients with cervical cancer – SEER data analysis. Head Neck 2008;30:58–66.
17 Kleinerman RA, Boice JD, Storm HH, et al: Second primary cancer after treatment for cervical cancer. Cancer 1995;76:442–452.
18 Ohno T, Kato S, Sato S, et al: Long-term survival and risk of second cancers after radiotherapy for cervical cancer. Int J Radiat Oncol Biol Phys 2007;69: 740–745.
19 Ota T, Takeshima N, Tabata T, et al: Treatment of squamous cell carcinoma of the uterine cervix with radiation therapy alone: long-term survival, late complications, and incidence of second cancers. Br J Cancer 2007;97:1058–1062.
20 Ohno T, Kakinuma S, Kato S, et al: Risk of second cancers after radiotherapy for cervical cancer. Exp Rev Anticancer Ther 2006;6:49–57.

Krueger H, McLean D, Williams D: The Prevention of Second Primary Cancers.
Prog Exp Tumor Res. Basel, Karger, 2008, vol 40, pp 111–121

13

Skin Cancers

The investigation of the major forms of skin cancer with respect to SPC risk may be characterized as intensive. The interest partly flows from the high prevalence (with respect to nonmelanoma skin cancer) or premature mortality (with respect to melanoma) of the first primary tumor, as well as the wide range of SPCs observed in cancer registries around the world [1].

Overall excess SPC risks following skin cancer have sometimes been evaluated as marginal. The most recent large epidemiologic profile revealed the same significant SIR of 1.2 in both men and women [2]. Other studies have offered even more modest results. For instance, an investigation of nonmelanoma skin cancer cases during a 45-year period in Manitoba suggested a SIR for all second cancers of 1.06 (95% CI 1.02–1.10) in men and 1.07 (95% CI 1.02–1.12) in women [3].

Within the overall statistics, however, we do find more sizeable SPC risks following tumors in particular epithelial tissues. The classic distinction in skin oncology is made between nonmelanoma and melanoma cancers. Nonmelanoma includes the 2 most common skin cancers – basal cell carcinoma and squamous cell carcinoma.

A 2004 investigation of 92,658 postmenopausal women offered the most extensive look at the combined category of nonmelanoma skin cancer [4]. The results that stand out in table 62 include the excess risk for second cancer of lung, breast, stomach and thyroid gland, as well as for leukemia, lymphoma and melanoma.

Apart from the bias involved with limiting the sample to older women, 1 problem with this study's cross-sectional approach (as opposed to using cancer registry data) is that a temporal relationship could not be established between skin cancer and the other cancers (this is why the table is entitled 'other primary cancer' rather than SPC). Confirming directionality requires a different study design. Addressing another methodological concern, it would be preferable to access research that does not combine tissue types, but rather looks at squamous cell and basal cell carcinomas as separate entities. This is because the SPC story related to different skin cancers demonstrates great variety.

Table 62. Other primary cancer associated with non-melanoma skin cancer

Other primary cancer	Overall SIR
Lung	3.43 (2.51–4.69)
Colorectal	1.68 (1.38–2.04)
Breast	2.09 (1.93–2.26)
NHL	2.73 (1.92–3.86)
Ovary	2.01 (1.61–2.50)
Brain	2.12 (1.02–4.39)
Leukemia	3.58 (2.21–5.80)
Stomach	3.17 (1.63–6.18)
Melanoma, skin	3.29 (2.87–3.76)
Cervix	1.92 (1.62–2.28)
Uterus	2.00 (1.74–2.29)
Thyroid gland	2.60 (2.07–3.28)
Hodgkin's disease	5.69 (3.12–10.39)
Liver	5.96 (2.71–13.11)
Bone	2.90 (1.55–5.44)
All cancers [5]	**2.30 (2.18–2.44)**

Figures in parentheses are 95% CI. Adapted from Rosenberg et al. [4].

Squamous Cell Carcinoma

Squamous cell carcinoma is the second most common nonmelanoma skin cancer after basal cell carcinoma. Squamous cell carcinoma has a higher rate of systemic spread compared to basal cell carcinoma. The largest investigation of SPC following cutaneous squamous cell carcinoma was conducted in 1999. The results for the almost 26,000 cases are summarized in table 63 [6].

While there is some overlap with the main nonmelanoma cancer associations in the cross-sectional study noted earlier, there are a number of differences. The most distinctive deletions from the list are breast and thyroid gland cancer, whereas the additions include malignancies of the oral cavity, nasopharynx, hypopharynx, salivary gland and lip. An association with lip cancer probably reflects a common carcinogen, namely, UV light. HPV may have a causal association with squamous cell carcinomas, thus explaining the connection to oral and pharyngeal cancers, where viral infection also plays a role. Several SPC sites show a more moderate SIR compared to table 62, notably the lung, stomach and liver. Another important implication of the study is the lack of a therapy effect, a result confirmed by other researchers.

Table 63. SPC following squamous cell carcinoma of the skin by follow-up period

SPC	Overall SIR	Years of follow-up: SIR			
		<1 year	1–4 years	5–9 years	10–14 years
Lung	1.7 (1.5–1.9)	2.2	1.7	1.8	
Colon	1.2 (1.1–1.4)	1.4	1.3		
NHL	1.9 (1.6–2.3)	2.8	2.2		
Lymphatic leukemia	1.8 (1.4–2.3)	2.1	2.4		
Myeloid leukemia	2.0 (1.4–2.7)		2.7		
Esophagus	1.5 (1.1–2.0)		1.7	1.9	
Stomach	1.3 (1.1–1.4)		1.4	1.4	
Oral	2.0 (1.2–3.2)	3.2			
Nasopharynx	3.0 (1.2–6.2)			5.4	
Hypopharynx	2.7 (1.5–4.7)			4.4	
Melanoma, skin	3.0 (2.5–3.7)	3.9	3.3	2.9	
Cervix	2.2 (1.4–3.2)		2.6		
Hodgkin's disease	2.1 (1.2–3.2)		3.3		
Liver and intrahepatic bile duct	1.3 (1.1–1.5)		1.5		
Vulva and vagina	2.3 (1.4–3.5)		2.4		4.2
Salivary gland	5.5 (3.7–8.0)		11.0		
Lip	5.2 (4.2–6.3)	4.4	5.8	6.4	4.1
Nonmelanoma skin cancer	15.6 (15.0–16.3)	22.9	17.2	13.4	11.6
All cancers	**2.2 (2.1–2.2)**				

Figures in parentheses are 95% CI. Adapted from Wassberg et al. [6].

Another large study looked at both in situ and invasive squamous cell carcinoma [7]. The results for SPC following invasive skin tumors (n = 17,637) are provided in table 64. There is a strong overlap with the data in table 63, notwithstanding the fact that the significant results in aerodigestive and digestive tissues are here specifically restricted to men. Considering etiologic linkages, smoking has been put forward by different researchers as the common causative agent explaining the excess risk of many SPCs following squamous cell cancer of the skin [2, 6]. That very factor (combined with UV exposure) has been proposed particularly for lip cancer, which often shows up in excess following squamous cell carcinoma. However, it must be acknowledged that contradictory evidence exists concerning the implications of smoking for the incidence of skin cancer itself [8, 9].

We note the strong showing again in this research for second salivary gland cancer, and the unusual risk in women for cancer related to the nose (consistent with the result for nasopharynx in the previous study). The same authors examined another set of data and found a similar result for the salivary gland; indeed, they remarked that there has

Table 64. SPC following invasive squamous cell carcinoma

SPC	Overall SIR	
	men	women
Lung	1.8 (1.5–2.0)	
NHL	1.7 (1.3–2.1)	
Stomach	1.3 (1.1–1.6)	
Kidney	1.5 (1.2–1.9)	
Oral	2.6 (2.1–3.2)	3.0 (1.9–4.5)
Nose		6.9 (2.2–14.4)
Melanoma, skin	2.0 (1.5–2.6)	2.3 (1.6–3.3)
Connective tissue	2.6 (1.6–4.0)	
Salivary gland	5.2 (2.8–8.4)	6.4 (2.5–12.1)
Nonmelanoma skin cancer	10.0 (9.4–10.7)	9.0 (7.9–10.2)
All cancers	**1.9 (1.8–1.9)**	**1.5 (1.4–1.7)**

Figures in parentheses are 95% CI. Adapted from Hemminki and Dong [7].

been an excess of salivary gland cancers in at least 6 other studies of squamous cell carcinoma of the skin [10]. Considering the 2 unique sites of the salivary gland and nose has led to the hypothesis that Epstein-Barr virus or other viral infection may be a common factor. In addition to malignancies of the salivary gland and the nasopharynx, Epstein-Barr virus has been implicated in lymphoma and in cancers of the stomach.

The same research team has provided evidence of a link between skin cancer and HPV-related cancers such as oral cancer [11]. Interestingly, HPV has also been proposed as an etiologic factor in salivary gland cancer [6].

While the role of Epstein-Barr virus and HPV remains speculative, it is likely that any such agents would not be acting in an 'environmental vacuum'. The usual biological context proposed for viral influence on carcinogenesis is immunosuppression. There is a growing understanding that sun exposure produces an immunosuppressed condition, in turn possibly accounting for various skin cancers [12]. This may lead to a variety of SPC implications. For instance, there has been strong evidence linking UV-related immunosuppression and the risk of NHL following skin cancer [13, 14]. Other immunocompromised populations, such as those receiving organ transplants, have demonstrated a similar pattern [4].

The preceding discussion may be summed up in terms of the 2 main prevention opportunities with respect to SPC, namely, smoking cessation and sun protection. Furthermore, as polyvalent HPV vaccines become more prevalent, any SPC caused by that viral infection may very well diminish.

Table 65. SPC following squamous cell skin cancer

SPC	Overall SIR
Pancreas	3.3 (1.2–9.1)
Genitourinary organs	1.5 (1.1–2.0)
Basal cell carcinoma	13.3 (8.5–20.6)
All cancers	**1.4 (1.2–1.7)**

Figures in parentheses are 95% CI. Adapted from Efird et al. [23].

We cannot leave the topic of sun protection without highlighting the current discussion around a countervailing mechanism proposed for UV exposure and its impact on vitamin D generation. Vitamin D seems to reduce the risk of several solid cancers, including stomach, colorectal, liver and gallbladder, pancreas, lung, female breast, prostate, bladder and kidney [15]. Of this list, mortality due to cancer of the prostate, colon and breast appears to be especially reduced with UV exposure [16, 17]. For example, a 2007 study of about 13,500 skin cancer patients established a SIR of 0.89 (95% CI 0.78–0.99) for second prostate tumors [18]. It is presumed that skin cancer is a proxy for both cumulative UV exposure and healthy levels of vitamin D production, leading to a protective effect in terms of cancer development. Interestingly, the colon and the female breast, though not the prostate, appear to be sites of elevated risk for SPC following skin cancer in certain epidemiologic reports (see above), which goes against the claims for vitamin D-related protection. This reflects only part of the controversy around this area of oncology and public health. The complexity extends to topics that were once considered well established. For instance, the possibility of a decreased rather than an increased incidence of NHL has recently been linked to sun exposure [19, 20]. Part of the challenge relates to the difficulty in measuring solar exposure in epidemiologic studies; proxies such as skin cancers, latitude, sunny climates, etc. are subject to confounding factors [21]. At the very least, the uncertainty suggests that any claim that the health benefits of sunlight outweigh the cancer risks are at least premature.

Finally, it is important to note the role of nonmelanoma skin cancer following cutaneous squamous cell carcinoma. Often the highest MPC risk is cutaneous squamous cell carcinoma itself, though arguably this does not count as a true SPC. Basal cell carcinomas also appear to show up in excess. A subset of cancer registries do include cases of basal cell carcinoma, and distinguish them from squamous cell types. A meta-analysis of the relevant literature up to 2000 indicated a 10-fold increase in the risk of contracting basal cell carcinoma after squamous cell cancer of the skin [22]. A smaller study from 2002 pegged the rate even higher (table 65) [23].

Table 66. SPC following basal cell carcinoma

SPC	Overall SIR	
	<60 years of age	≥60 years of age
Breast	1.37 (1.09–1.70)	
NHL	2.50 (1.60–3.72)	
Leukemia		1.41 (1.15–1.72)
Melanoma, skin	3.22 (2.33–4.34)	2.44 (1.96–2.99)
Testis	3.52 (1.61–6.68)	
Hodgkin's disease		2.17 (1.08–3.88)
Lip	2.71 (1.10–5.65)	1.97 (1.34–2.77)
All cancers	**1.26 (1.16–1.37)**	**1.11 (1.07–1.14)**

Figures in parentheses are 95% CI. Adapted from Frisch et al. [25].

Although not reflected in the study just noted, data from other research suggest an elevated risk for melanoma skin cancer following squamous cell carcinoma. The traditional linkage suggested has once again been UV radiation exposure, but recent analysis also points to the role of genetic susceptibility [7]. Indeed, the impact of inherent genetic defects (for example, a reduced ability to repair DNA damage) on SPC following squamous cell carcinomas is just beginning to be investigated [24].

Basal Cell Carcinoma

The most common form of skin cancer in Caucasian populations is basal cell carcinoma. It occurs at such a high rate that, bizarrely, it is often not included in cancer registries. Nonetheless, the results from an older study (table 66) confirm that there is a demonstrable excess risk for a limited range of SPCs [25]. Most cancers of interest match the pattern following squamous cell skin cancer. These include lymphomas, leukemia, melanoma and cancer of the lip. While not reflected here, there is also a well-known increased risk of squamous cell carcinoma following basal cell carcinomas.

The same lead author produced a much larger population-based study (n = 37,674) a couple of years later [26]. The additional SPCs of excess risk observed there included malignancies of the salivary gland, kidney and upper aerodigestive tract. Another 1998 study (n = 11,878) confirmed significant SIRs for lip cancer, NHL and melanoma following basal cell carcinoma [27]. A good approach to understanding such associations involves the same etiologic factors introduced in our discussion of first primary squamous cell carcinoma.

Table 67. SPC following basal cell carcinoma (2 studies indicated by lead author)

SPC	Overall SIR			
	men		women	
	Friedman	Milan	Friedman	Milan
Lung	1.90	1.13		
Colon		1.30		1.23
Rectum		1.17		
Breast				1.23
NHL		1.37		1.48
Prostate		1.22		
Leukemia		1.50		1.24
Stomach				1.17
Kidney		1.23	2.30	
Oral		1.69		
Nose and sinus		1.88		
Pharynx		1.67		1.75
Urinary bladder		1.17		
Melanoma, skin	2.10	2.39	2.20	2.30
Multiple myeloma		1.45		
Liver		1.40		
Small intestine		1.82		1.88
Eye				1.91
Nervous system		1.34		1.33
Salivary gland		4.28		2.49
Bone		2.06		
Lip		2.07		2.58
Nonmelanoma skin cancer		4.05		3.59
All cancers	**1.20**	**1.32**	**1.20**	**1.30**

Adapted from Milan et al. [28] and Friedman and Tekawa [29].

Unlike other cancer topics with very recent research results, the most substantial work for basal cell carcinoma seems to date back to 2000. For a comparison of statistical power and different research approaches, we have placed 2 older papers side by side, a population analysis by Milan et al. [28] (n = 71,924) and a retrospective study by Friedman and Tekawa [29] (n = 3,164). In the interest of space, we have not included each 95% CI, but in all cases presented here the interval did not include unity, that is, they were statistically significant (table 67).

Not surprisingly, the larger study produced a wider range of associations. The key overlap with the study by Friedman and Tekawa relates to melanoma skin cancer as a second primary. In the end, the most interesting result is that both studies revealed a

Table 68. SPC following cutaneous melanoma

Secondary Primary Cancer	Overall SIR (95% CI)	
	men	women
Kidney	3.5 (1.4–7.2)	
Melanoma	38.5 (30.4–48.1)	29.0 (22.0–37.5)

Adapted from: Schmid-Wendtner et al. [33].

modest SIR for all SPCs. Yet another study, larger than that of Friedman and Tekawa, was even more conservative. The results of a British cancer registry investigation (n = 13,961 cases of basal cell carcinoma) showed an excess risk of SPC only for melanoma [30]. One reason for what might be perceived as a relatively low interest in basal cell carcinoma as an antecedent condition to other cancers is the relatively low excess incidence of second primaries as a class.

Melanoma

The dominant message concerning SPC following skin melanoma is the fact that there is little evidence of excess risk, outside of skin cancers themselves. It is well established that both basal cell and squamous cell carcinomas have a higher incidence following melanoma [31, 32].

Multiple primary melanomas represent a whole field of study on their own, for reasons that are made clear in table 68. The results summarized there, based on a moderately sized prospective study in 2001 (n = 4,597 melanoma patients), demonstrate a dramatic risk of multiple melanomas [33]. What is most startling about this table is the fact that there are no other significant associations apart from kidney cancer in men. This result has been confirmed in a remarkable range of studies over a 10-year period [27, 34–36]. Indeed, in some studies there is a deficiency of certain SPCs, with an explanation for such a protective effect still lacking.

The one exception to this analysis may be NHL. In a 2004 review of 1,835 melanoma cases, Crocetti and Carli [37] identified a SIR of 2.74 for NHL as a second cancer, but the result barely achieved statistical significance (95% CI 1.01–5.94). Earlier studies have demonstrated SIRs modestly above unity, both significant and nonsignificant [38, 39]. A substantial pooled analysis was completed in 2005. Lens and Newton-Bishop [40] reviewed 109,532 cutaneous melanoma cases in the literature

Table 69. SPC following Merkel cell carcinoma

SPC	Overall SIR
NHL	2.56 (1.23–4.71)
Biliary other than liver and gallbladder	7.24 (1.46–21.16)
Salivary gland	11.55 (2.32–33.76)
All cancers	**1.22 (1.01–1.45)**

Figures in parentheses are 95% CI. Adapted from Howard et al. [41].

up to 2004, concluding that the SIR for NHL was 2.01 (95% CI 1.79–2.24). The proposed common risk factors will be familiar from our discussion of squamous cell carcinoma, namely, the mutagenic and immunosuppressive effects of UV exposure and possibly the influence of genetic inheritance. There is also a hypothesis that implicates immunodeficiency mechanisms mediated by melanoma itself.

Based on current information, the prevention bottom line for SPC following cutaneous melanoma, apart from surveillance for new skin cancers, is the well-known proviso of broad-spectrum sun protection.

Merkel Cell Carcinoma

As seen with other topics in this monograph, where the research related to SPC appears to be reaching a 'mature' point, the recent work around skin cancer has moved into specialty topics. Thus, a study from late 2006 examined the SPC risk following cases (n = 1,306) of Merkel cell carcinoma, a rare neuroendocrine cancer of the skin [41]. It revealed a few significant and substantial associations (table 69).

The etiologic mechanisms related to the elevated SPC risks remain under investigation. Of special interest is the possible biological overlap with other small cell and neuroendocrine tumors of, for instance, the salivary gland.

Notes and References

1 See, for example, the results in Troyanova P, Danon S, Ivanova T: Nonmelanoma skin cancers and risk of subsequent malignancies: a cancer registry-based study in Bulgaria. Neoplasma 2002;49:81–85.

2 Maitra SK, Gallo H, Rowland-Payne C, et al: Second primary cancers in patients with squamous cell carcinoma of the skin. Br J Cancer 2005;92:570–571.

3 Nugent Z, Demers AA, Wiseman MC, et al: Risk of second primary cancer and death following a diagnosis of nonmelanoma skin cancer. Cancer Epidemiol Biomarkers Prev 2005;14:2584–2590.

4 Rosenberg CA, Greenland P, Khandekar J, et al: Association of nonmelanoma skin cancer with second malignancy. Cancer 2004;100:130–138.

5 Excluding nonmelanoma skin cancer.
6 Wassberg C, Thorn M, Yuen J, et al: Second primary cancers in patients with squamous cell carcinoma of the skin: a population-based study in Sweden. Int J Cancer 1999;80:511–515.
7 Hemminki K, Dong C: Subsequent cancers after in situ and invasive squamous cell carcinoma of the skin. Arch Dermatol 2000;136:647–651.
8 Grodstein F, Speizer FE, Hunter DJ: A prospective study of incident squamous cell carcinoma of the skin in the nurses' health study. J Natl Cancer Inst 1996; 88:56.
9 Odenbro A, Bellocco R, Boffetta P, et al: Tobacco smoking, snuff dipping and the risk of cutaneous squamous cell carcinoma: a nationwide cohort study in Sweden. Br J Cancer 2005;92:1326–1328.
10 Hemminki K, Dong C: Primary cancers following squamous cell carcinoma of the skin suggest involvement of Epstein-Barr virus. Epidemiology 2000;11:94.
11 Hemminki K, Jiang Y, Dong C: Second primary cancers after anogenital, skin, oral, esophageal and rectal cancers: etiological links? Int J Cancer 2001;93: 294–298.
12 Parrish J: Immunosuppression, skin cancer and ultraviolet A radiation. N Engl J Med 2005;353:2712–2713.
13 Hemminki K, Jiang Y, Steineck G: Skin cancer and non-Hodgkin's lymphoma as second malignancies: markers of impaired immune function? Eur J Cancer 2003;39:223–229.
14 Hall P, Rosendahl I, Mattsson A, et al: Non-Hodgkin's lymphoma and skin malignancies – shared etiology? Int J Cancer 1995;62:519–522.
15 Tuohimaa P, Pukkala E, Scelo G, et al: Does solar exposure, as indicated by the non-melanoma skin cancers, protect from solid cancers: vitamin D as a possible explanation. Eur J Cancer 2007;43:1701–1712.
16 Krause R, Matulla-Nolte B, Essers M, et al: UV radiation and cancer prevention: what is the evidence? Anticancer Res 2006;26:2723–2727.
17 Osborne JE, Hutchinson PE: Vitamin D and systemic cancer: is this relevant to malignant melanoma? Br J Cancer 2002;147:197–213.
18 De Vries E, Soerjomataram I, Houterman S, et al: Decreased risk of prostate cancer after skin cancer diagnosis: a protective role of ultraviolet radiation? Am J Epidemiol 2007;165:966–972.
19 Armstrong BK, Kricker A: Sun exposure and non-Hodgkin lymphoma. Cancer Epidemiol Biomarkers Prev 2007;16:396–400.
20 Kricker A, Armstrong BK, Hughes AM, et al: Personal sun exposure and risk of non Hodgkin lymphoma: a pooled analysis from the Interlymph Consortium. Int J Cancer 2008;122:144–154.
21 Grimsrud TK, Andersen A: Protective effect from solar exposure, risk of an ecological fallacy. Eur J Cancer 2008;44:16–18.
22 Marcil I, Stern RS: Risk of developing a subsequent nonmelanoma skin cancer in patients with a history of nonmelanoma skin cancer: a critical review of the literature and meta-analysis. Arch Dermatol 2000;136: 1524–1530.
23 Efird JT, Friedman GD, Habel L, et al: Risk of subsequent cancer following invasive or in situ squamous cell skin cancer. Ann Epidemiol 2002;12:469–475.
24 Brewster AM, Alberg AJ, Strickland PT, et al: XPB polymorphism and risk of subsequent cancer in individuals with nonmelanoma skin cancer. Cancer Epidemiol Biomarkers Prev 2004;13:1271–1275.
25 Frisch M, Hjalgrim H, Olsen JH, et al: Risk for subsequent cancer after diagnosis of basal-cell carcinoma: a population-based, epidemiologic study. Ann Intern Med 1996;125:815–821.
26 Frisch M, Hjalgrim H, Olsen JH, et al: Risk of cancer among patients with cutaneous basal cell carcinoma. Ugeskr Laeger 1998;160:2882–2887.
27 Levi F, La Vecchia C, Te VC, et al: Incidence of invasive cancers following basal cell skin cancer. Am J Epidemiol 1998;147:722–726.
28 Milan T, Pukkala E, Verkasalo PK, et al: Subsequent primary cancers after basal-cell carcinoma: a nationwide study in Finland from 1953 to 1995. Int J Cancer 2000;87:283–288.
29 Friedman GD, Tekawa IS: Association of basal cell skin cancers with other cancers (United States). Cancer Causes Control 2000;11:891–897. Note that the results provided were based on multivariate analysis rather than crude data.
30 Bower CP, Lear JT, Bygrave S, et al: Basal cell carcinoma and risk of subsequent malignancies: a cancer registry-based study in southwest England. J Am Acad Dermatol 2000;42:988–991.
31 Kroumpouzos G, Konstadoulakis MM, Cabral H, et al: Risk of basal cell and squamous cell carcinoma in persons with prior cutaneous melanoma. Dermatol Surg 2000;26:547–550.
32 Neale RE, Forman D, Murphy MF, et al: Site-specific occurrence of nonmelanoma skin cancers in patients with cutaneous melanoma. Br J Cancer 2005;93: 597–601.
33 Schmid-Wendtner MH, Baumert J, Wendtner CM, et al: Risk of second primary malignancies in patients with cutaneous melanoma. Br J Dermatol 2001;145: 981–985.
34 Schenk M, Severson RK, Pawlish KS: The risk of subsequent primary carcinoma of the pancreas in patients with cutaneous malignant melanoma. Cancer 1998;82: 1672–1676.
35 Bhatia S, Estrada-Batres L, Maryon T, et al: Second primary tumors in patients with cutaneous malignant melanoma. Cancer 1999;86:2014–2020.

36 Wu Y, Kim GH, Wagner JD, et al: The association between malignant melanoma and noncutaneous malignancies. Int J Dermatol 2006;45:529–534.
37 Crocetti E, Carli P: Risk of second primary cancers, other than melanoma, in an Italian population-based cohort of cutaneous malignant melanoma patients. Eur J Cancer Prev 2004;13:33–37.
38 Goggins WB, Finelstein DM, Tsao H: Evidence for an association between cutaneous melanoma and non-Hodgkin lymphoma. Cancer 2001;91:874–880.
39 McKenna DB, Stockton D, Brewster DH, et al: Evidence for an association between cutaneous malignant melanoma and lymphoid malignancy: a population-based retrospective cohort study in Scotland. Br J Cancer 2003;88:74–78.
40 Lens MB, Newton-Bishop JA: An association between cutaneous melanoma and non-Hodgkin's lymphoma: pooled analysis of published data with a review. Ann Oncol 2005;16:460–465.
41 Howard RA, Dores GM, Curtis RE, et al: Merkel cell carcinoma and multiple primary cancers. Cancer Epidemiol Biomarkers Prev 2006;15:1545–1549.

Krueger H, McLean D, Williams D: The Prevention of Second Primary Cancers.
Prog Exp Tumor Res. Basel, Karger, 2008, vol 40, pp 122–134

14

Pediatric Cancers

As we introduced in chapter 3 (pp 17–24), pediatric first primary cancers are of particular interest as predictors of increased risk for a subsequent malignancy. We also noted that 4 pediatric cancers dominate the research in this area. In this chapter, we will mainly review the information available for SPC following Hodgkin's disease, acute lymphocytic leukemia, retinoblastoma and Wilms tumor presenting in the pediatric age group.

Knowing the specific SPCs in excess following particular types of pediatric cancer is generally of more precise clinical utility than the aggregate risk information provided in chapter 3 (pp 17–24). On the other hand, pooled data across all childhood cancer survivors has permitted modeling that predicts the volume of SPCs of different types, which might allow for surveillance and treatment resource planning in certain jurisdictions [1]. This sort of population level benefit continues to drive research that treats pediatric first primaries as a class [2–6]. One fact that continues to emerge from combined studies is the overwhelming importance of therapy, and especially radiation, as a cause of excess cases of a variety of SPCs [7–10]. The largest recent analysis combining data across pediatric cancer cases (n = 25,965) was based on the US SEER database [11]. Table 70 contains all significant results.

However important the details may be, the overall conclusion from these data is that SPC following pediatric cancer is a serious public health concern. Indeed, a US study revealed that SPC was the leading cause of death after 15 years of follow-up of childhood cancer survivors [12]. Recent follow-up guidelines have situated cancer prevention and surveillance on the broader agenda of follow-up among child and adolescent survivors of cancer [13, 14]. We will now address the more targeted prevention and surveillance concerns that are attached to particular pediatric first primaries.

Hodgkin's Disease

The introduction of combination therapy in the mid-1960s has produced a 10-year survival rate of 90% for children with Hodgkin's disease. As we might now expect at

Table 70. SPC following pediatric cancers by follow-up period

SPC	Overall SIR	Years of follow-up: SIR					
		≤1 year	1–4 years	5–9 years	10–14 years	15–19 years	≥20 years
Lung	7.4				15.7		
Colorectal	3.9			16.4			
Breast	8.4				15.1	11.8	5.0
Pancreas	24.7		117.4			54.3	
NHL	3.5	9.9		4.9			4.3
Brain	7.9	6.8	4.6	10.7	9.2	6.9	11.0
Prostate	14.9			113.6			
Leukemia							
Acute lymphocytic leukemia	2.2						
Acute myeloid leukemia	17.1		45.1	14.2	7.6		
Chronic myeloid leukemia	5.1		21.2				
Esophagus	23.8						
Stomach	17.0					32.6	24.1
Kidney	4.5					12.0	
Nose and sinus	11.6			52.9			
Oral/pharynx	13.0		10.7	15.7	20.9	14.5	
Melanoma, skin	4.0	54.4	6.6	5.4	3.4		
Uterus	6.2						
Thyroid	6.7		6.4	8.3	8.7	4.8	5.1
Testis	2.1		8.4				
Small intestine	29.1		108.6				
Eye	13.1	21.0					
Soft tissue	14.1		9.5	19.9	13.3	24.1	
Salivary gland	20.5			20.9	29.9	24.8	
Bone	18.6		18.6	19.0	18.2	18.2	39.2
Mesothelioma	55.5					107.1	89.6
All cancers	**5.9**	**6.1**	**7.7**	**7.6**	**5.5**	**5.1**	**4.1**

Adapted from Inskip and Curtis [11].

Table 71. SPC following pediatric Hodgkin's disease by follow-up period

SPC	Overall SIR	Years of follow-up: SIR			
		5–9 years	10–14 years	15–19 years	≥20 years
Lung	5.1 (1.9–11.1)				
Colorectal					
Colon	4.7 (1.3–12.1)				
Rectum	12.4 (4.0–28.9)				
Breast (female)	14.1 ($p<0.05$)	9.7	25.7	18.4	8.0
Pancreas	10.8 (1.2–38.9)				
NHL	6.9 (3.3–12.8)				
Leukemia	20.9 (13.9–30.3)				
All acute	27.4 (17.9–40.2)				
Esophagus	65.3 (17.6–167.0)				
Stomach	13.8 (4.4–32.1)				
Cervix	6.1 ($p<0.05$)		10.5	5.3	10.3
Thyroid gland	13.7 (8.6–20.7)	6.5	22.7	12.0	37.7
Sarcomas		6.3	20.0	43.0	10.6
Connective tissue	15.1 (6.9–28.7)				
Bone	9.7 (3.1–22.7)				

Figures in parentheses are 95% CI, unless indicated otherwise. Adapted from Metayer et al. [15].

this point in the monograph, a long survival period raises the possibility of late effects developing, including SPC. This is especially a concern among patients from past decades who were subject to aggressive (and often successful) therapies.

Table 71 was adapted from a 2000 study by Metayer et al. [15], which was based on a sample of almost 6,000 survivors of Hodgkin's disease diagnosed before age 21.

How do these data stand up against other studies? Lin and Teitell [16] offer a helpful review of the literature up to 2004. As an example, the SIR for lung cancer after pediatric Hodgkin's disease ranged from 5.1 to 27.3 (similar to the experience seen in adult-onset Hodgkin's disease); furthermore, the risk increased after 10–15 years (consistent with other solid tumors following Hodgkin's disease). The wider literature supports the significant excess of other solid tumors recorded in the table, including those of the gastrointestinal tract, breast, cervix, bone and connective tissue as well as thyroid gland. A lower risk is confirmed for male genital tract SPC compared to female genital and urinary tract tumors. Furthermore, neurologic SPC is confirmed as being rare, while excess melanoma (influenced by chemotherapy) may be more

Table 72. SPC following pediatric Hodgkin's disease

SPC	Overall SIR
Lung	23.7 (2.87–85.6)
Breast	20.9 (7.66–45.4)
Pancreas	44.4 (1.11–247)
Brain	7.76 (1.60–22.7)
Leukemia	
Myeloid leukemia	33.9 (9.24–86.8)
Other leukemia	53.7 (17.4–125)
Melanoma, skin	6.71 (1.38–19.6)
Thyroid	52.5 (24.0–99.6)
Soft tissue sarcoma	17.8 (2.16–64.4)
Other male genital	142 (3.56–794)
Nonmelanoma skin	34.0 (12.5–74.0)
All cancers	**12.4 (9.12–16.4)**

Figures in parentheses are 95% CI. Adapted from Maule et al. [18].

substantial than suggested by Metayer and colleagues. Some research updates suggest additions to the list. For instance, the recent analysis by Bhatia et al. [17] revealed that thyroid cancer might be the second most common solid tumor (after breast cancer) in these pediatric Hodgkin's disease survivors.

The latest research evaluated a relatively small pool of Hodgkin's disease cases (n = 1,246), but had the advantage of being drawn from 13 cancer registries from different parts of the world [18]. As table 72 shows, the study reproduced the key categories of excess SPC detected by Metayer and colleagues, with the exception of colorectal cancer.

Specific SPCs have received special attention in the literature. As noted earlier in the monograph, there has been controversy about the statistical methods used to track increases in SPC of the breast over longer follow-up. Although it does not seem to be supported by the data in the study by Metayer and coauthors, most investigators agree that incidence rises 10–20 years after successful Hodgkin's disease therapy, that is, among women between 30 and 40 years. This is 20 or more years earlier than the general population, consistent with the experience of familial cases of breast cancer involving *BRCA1* and *BRCA2* mutations. The suggestion is that a premalignant state is present in children cured of Hodgkin's disease, and that this premalignant state has a strong treatment-related component (see below).

Leukemia is well documented as one of the most common malignant late effects in both pediatric and adult Hodgkin's disease. The SIR in childhood cancer survivors has been recorded to be as high as 175. NHL is also a commonly occurring malignancy subsequent to Hodgkin's disease, with the reported SIR being between 5 and 20.

The discussion of etiology and preventive measures will be based on the review by Lin and Teitell [16]. First, acute leukemia is strongly associated with chemotherapy for Hodgkin's disease, especially alkylating agents such as cyclophosphamide and epipodophyllotoxins such as etoposide. One study underlined the latter association, suggesting a dose-dependent effect on leukemia risk. Another study demonstrated that limiting cumulative doses of alkylating agent therapy and avoiding especially risky agents, such as mechlorethamine, led to a decline in leukemia incidence [19].

While risk factors for NHL have yet to be defined, there is the suggestion that an immunocompromised state may be involved, and possibly an infectious agent such as the Epstein-Barr virus.

Although the evidence for chemotherapy is mixed, radiation to treat Hodgkin's disease is less equivocal; it has been strongly linked to second primary breast cancer, which often presents bilaterally. Radiation therapy during puberty and young adulthood is associated with increased risk, suggesting that the breast may be in 'an ovarian hormone-sensitive, proliferative state that is more sensitive to carcinogenic effects'. Similarly, any conditions that affect ovarian hormone levels may have an impact on the risk of SPC of the breast. Radiation dose seems to be an important factor. A recent study [17] showed that no excess breast tumors developed when the therapy dosage was kept below the current recommended exposure limit of 26 Gy [20].

The etiology of second primary lung cancer is still being uncovered. Radiation and chemotherapy effects seem to be additive. Although causing less concern than in cases involving adult Hodgkin's disease treatment, smoking is a significant risk factor subsequent to therapy, and provides an obvious candidate for preventive efforts.

Radiation-induced damage is strongly implicated in gastrointestinal SPC, and may even be a necessary cause. Unfortunately, cancer often begins without symptoms so that most second primary tumors present at advanced, aggressive stages. So far, there have been no studies confirming the optimum time to begin screening, though one guideline recommends 10 years after radiation or at age 35 (whichever occurs last) [21].

The suggestion in the case of SPC of the cervix is that Hodgkin's disease may induce defective cellular immunity that in turn causes the carcinogenic impact of HPV infection to be more serious. Chemotherapy, but not radiotherapy, may amplify such conditions. Encouraging healthy sexual practice would be an appropriate preventive intervention, though obviously such measures are motivated by rationales far beyond the care regimen for pediatric Hodgkin's disease. HPV vaccination in adolescent survivors of cancer may ultimately be very useful in this regard.

The sensitivity of the thyroid gland to radiation-induced damage is well established [22]. For instance, Bhatia et al. [17] found that 95% of tumors in the thyroid were confined to the radiation field. No primary prevention responses have yet been suggested by authorities, but regular clinical assessment at least is indicated.

To sum up, the best hope for SPC prevention following pediatric Hodgkin's disease seems to be therapy-related, specifically any strategy to detect Hodgkin's disease at an earlier stage where less intensive chemotherapy is effective and radiation therapy may be avoided altogether [23, 24]. From the point of view of second breast cancer development in particular, any treatments instituted prior to puberty appear to be manifestly safer.

Acute Lymphocytic Leukemia

Acute lymphocytic leukemia is the most common form of cancer in children, accounting for 25% of all pediatric malignancies. The peak incidence occurs in children from 2 to 5 years of age. Therapeutic advances have altered the outcome from routine mortality to a 5-year survival rate approaching 80% [25]. Treatments include chemotherapy and sometimes cranial irradiation. As one review noted, 'the recognition that [acute lymphocytic leukemia] is a heterogeneous disease and that children can be stratified into various risk groups has profoundly influenced therapy and outcome' [26].

As in the case of other long-survival cancers, the incidence of SPC following acute lymphocytic leukemia is a growing concern. A 2004 literature review included with a case report noted 230 cases of SPC in 25,051 children treated for acute lymphocytic leukemia, for a cumulative incidence of about 1% [27]. Once again, this figure by itself is not that helpful, as it does not indicate excess risk. The analysis of 8,831 children from the Children's Cancer Group diagnosed with acute lymphocytic leukemia was more informative; it revealed a cumulative incidence of 1.18% (95% CI 0.8–1.5), which represented a SIR of 7.2 [28]. This may be compared with the study by Neglia et al. [29], who reported a SIR of 5.7 (95% CI 4.37–7.22) for SPC among 4,581 leukemia cases, and with the study by Kowalczyk et al. [30], who reported a SIR of 6.0 in a cohort of 3,252 children with various forms of leukemia. The best breakdown for individual types of SPC is offered by the same large cohort of acute lymphocytic leukemia survivors from the Children's Cancer Group noted above (table 73) [28].

These results may be compared to the results found in a large 2007 study of all types of first primary leukemias in children (n = 12,731) [18]. While table 74 demonstrates a larger range of excess SPCs, there is good consistency with the data specific to NHL, brain cancer and thyroid gland cancer.

A smaller 2007 study did generate data specific to acute lymphocytic leukemia, confirming a very high SIR for nonlymphocytic leukemia (SIR = 150.9, 95% CI 98.1–185.4), as well as elevated risk for lymphomas and central nervous system tumors. The SIR for all SPCs was 13.5 (95% CI 10.9–16.8), the highest seen among the studies we have cited [32]. Two other 2007 studies documented increased levels of meningioma following

Table 73. SPC following pediatric acute lymphocytic leukemia by follow-up period

SPCs	Overall SIR	Years of follow-up: SIR			
		0–5 years	6–10 years	11–15 years	≥20 years
NHL	8.3 (2.6–17.2)				
Brain/central nervous system	10.1 (5.9–16.2)	10.8 (2.8–24)	17.5 (8.7–29.3)		
Leukemia					
ANLL [35]	52.3 (28.6–87.7)	233.9 (137.9–350.5)	31.6 (5.9–77.4)		
Thyroid Gland	13.3 (3.6–34.1)				
Sarcomas					
Soft tissue	9.1 (2.5–20.2)				
Parotid gland	33.4 (9.1–85.6)				
All cancers	**7.2 (5.5–9.1)**	**20.6 (5.8–28.0)**	**6.1 (3.6–9.3)**	**2.3 (1.0–4.3)**	

Figures in parentheses are 95% CI. ANLL = Acute non-lymphocytic leukemia. Adapted from Bhatia et al. [28].

Table 74. SPC following pediatric leukemia

SPC	Overall SIR
NHL	9.4 (4.3–17.9)
Brain	8.5 (5.1–13.3)
Bladder	53.6 (14.6–137.0)
Thyroid	18.8 (8.6–35.7)
Hodgkin's disease	3.9 (1.1–9.9)
Liver	25.6 (3.0–89.0)
Tongue	71.9 (8.7–260.0)
Salivary gland	31.5 (3.8–114.0)
Bone	5.0 (1.04–14.7)
Nonmelanoma skin	14.3 (3.9–36.7)
All cancers	**6.1 (4.7–7.8)**

Figures in parentheses are 95% CI. Adapted from Maule et al. [18].

acute lymphocytic leukemia [33, 34]. However, acute nonlymphocytic leukemia remains the outstanding clinical and public health concern following acute lymphocytic leukemia.

Although safer therapeutic protocols are being developed that will benefit future patients [35], the main priority in SPC prevention in patients who have had acute lymphocytic leukemia continues to be surveillance guided by the particular therapeutic risk exposure during treatment. This means: (1) regular, complete blood counts after chemotherapy to detect the precursor condition leading to acute nonlymphocytic leukemia [36] and (2) monitoring for the late effects of any cranial irradiation (usually in the radiation field itself, for example, tumors in the brain or parotid gland) [37, 38]. Of the areas of concern, brain or central nervous system tumors should perhaps take precedence as they are the most common form of SPC subsequent to acute lymphocytic leukemia [35]. As risks of brain as well as head and neck cancers increase with radiation dose [28], there has been an understandable trend towards reducing or eliminating the use of cranial radiation whenever possible [26].

We should note that there are well-known genetic predispositions related to both radiation and chemotherapy risks following acute lymphocytic leukemia, but these do not yet have preventive significance outside of guiding surveillance [35].

Finally, care must be taken with the delivery and follow-up of immunosuppression regimens associated with the various forms of transplantation used to treat leukemia. The types of cancer known to occur after such therapies often involve viral triggers that operate with impunity in immunodeficient environments. Examples include HPV, leading to cervical and oropharyngeal cancers, and Epstein-Barr virus, implicated in lymphomas [39, 40].

Retinoblastoma

Retinoblastoma, a malignant tumor of the developing retina, is the most frequent intraocular tumor in early childhood. There has apparently been increasing incidence since the beginning of the 1900s, but recently the disease frequency stabilized at around 1 in 16,000 [41].

Retinoblastoma usually occurs before the age of 5, and may be bilateral (affecting both eyes) or unilateral [42]. The disease occurs in cells with cancer susceptibility due to a genetic mutation in both copies of the gene known as *RB1*. Indeed, this was the first tumor suppressor gene to be isolated by researchers [43], and, as such, 'has provided many insights that apply broadly to the entire field of cancer biology' [44]. Retinoblastoma has been of special clinical interest because, like Wilms tumor (see below), it occurs in both hereditary (familial) and sporadic forms. The heritable form involves a germline mutation [45] that is passed on by a parent, with a somatic change in the remaining wild-type *RB1* gene completing the transition to a disease condition. Classically, these patients demonstrate bilateral involvement of retinal cells, since the required somatic mutations actually happen with relatively high frequency. Unlike the hereditary form that begins with a genetic contribution from a parent, sporadic retinoblastoma involves somatic mutations occurring successively in both *RB1* alleles of a retinal cell. It is responsible for most cases of unilateral disease [46].

Modern management depends on conservative therapies aimed at preserving the eye, including chemotherapy followed by focal laser or cryotherapy [47]. The current cure rate is very high.

Those with hereditary retinoblastoma show an increased risk of developing other, nonocular tumors. A 1997 review identified 11 studies in the literature; it noted that there had been 35 different types of cancer among the 243 cases of SPC detected following retinoblastoma. The most common were osteosarcomas (37%), other sarcomas, melanomas (7.4%) and brain tumors (4.5%). The cumulative incidence was 8.4% at 18 years after diagnosis, and the SIR for all SPCs was 15.4 [48]. This compares with a 1998 study of 180 patients, where the cumulative incidence was 16% at 25 years and 30% at 40 years [49]. The cumulative risk of death from second cancer at 40 years after diagnosis has been reported as 26% [50]. A more recent investigation of British retinoblastoma survivors with less exposure to high-dose radiation therapy demonstrated higher risk for common epithelial cancers, especially in the lung and bladder, and possibly the breast, compared to sarcomas [46].

Overall, the incidence of SPC in these studies tends to be too small to ascertain accurate SIR measures. The most recent study that attempted to expand the knowledge base looked at 963 one-year survivors of retinoblastoma [51]. It found a notable excess risk of soft tissue sarcomas (especially leiomyosarcomas), with a SIR of 184 (95% CI 143–233).

Clearly, prevention efforts should begin with ascertaining the genetic status (for example, through molecular genetic testing) and offering appropriate genetic counseling to any person where familial risk is likely [52]. Essentially, a person carrying a germline mutation in the *RB1* tumor suppression gene encountering any DNA-damaging agent that can cause a mutation in the second *RB1* allele will experience increased risk for retinoblastoma as well as other cancers exacerbated by the same mutation. Thus, combined with inherited genetic propensity, radiation therapy is a major risk factor for certain SPCs following retinoblastoma [53]. For instance, one study has shown a dose-response relationship for all second primary sarcomas [54]. Because of the risk, radiation therapy is limited to the most resistant cases [47].

While tobacco smoking has been strongly implicated in the development of SPC of the lung and bladder, UV radiation is a known carcinogen for melanoma. There has been long-standing advice for hereditary retinoblastoma survivors to avoid tobacco use [44, 53]. Behaviors related to sun safety are also recommended.

Wilms Tumor

Wilms tumor, also called nephroblastoma, is a cancer of the kidney. It occurs in about 1 in 12,000 children, equating to approximately 450 new cases annually in North

Table 75. Summary of research on Wilms tumor and SPC

Lead researcher	Year published	Sample size	SIR
Li [57]	1983	412 [58]	15.7
Breslow [59]	1988	2,438	8.5 (4.7–14.0)
Breslow [60]	1995	5,278	8.4 (6.1–11.4)
Carli [61]	1997	1,988	4.2 (1.8–8.2)
Neglia [29]	2001	1,174	6.0 (3.4–10.0)
Inskip [11]	2007	1,277	5.3 ($p < 0.05$)

Figures in parentheses are 95% CI, unless indicated otherwise.

America. It is the second most common solid tumor outside the brain in children, constituting about 6–7% of all pediatric cancers. About 90% of all kidney cancers in children are Wilms tumor. It is most often diagnosed between the ages of 6 months and 10 years, with the greatest number of children diagnosed by age 5. Bilateral tumors (in both kidneys) tend to be discovered at younger ages compared with unilateral forms of the disease.

Wilms tumor parallels retinoblastoma in several ways. Both malignancies occur in the very young, involve paired organs, arise from embryonal cells, can develop unilaterally or bilaterally, and can occur in hereditary and nonhereditary forms.

As with many other childhood cancers, outcomes for Wilms tumor have dramatically improved in recent years. Five-year survival in 1979 was 33%; now it is 90% or higher [55, 56]. Children diagnosed with Wilms tumor usually have a nephrectomy before any other therapy is initiated. In most North American centers, only children with bilateral Wilms tumor receive chemotherapy prior to surgery. After surgery, it is common for children with Wilms tumor to receive chemotherapy as part of their treatment protocol. For those with more advanced stages of disease, external beam radiation therapy is also given.

The literature on SPC following Wilms tumor is not very extensive; information is especially scarce for metachronous bilateral tumors [55]. The most comprehensive data concerning Wilms tumor and second malignancies is 10–15 years old. Table 75 summarizes what is known about overall occurrence, including data from trials guided by the International Society of Pediatric Oncology in Europe and equivalent North American groups.

The results concerning excess second cancers have been reasonably consistent. Considered over the medium term, the cumulative 10-year risk for SPC subsequent to Wilms tumor is about 1%. The absolute number of cases related to SPC is so small that it is challenging to get a fix on specific types of subsequent cancer. Analysis of 43 SPC cases in North America revealed that about 25% were leukemia or lymphoma (with acute nonlymphocytic leukemia predominating) and 14% were sarcoma of the bone or cartilage [62].

There is strong circumstantial evidence for radiotherapy being implicated in SPC following Wilms tumor, including the possibility of a dose effect [57, 60, 63]. Most second neoplasms reported have occurred in irradiated areas. This includes colorectal adenocarcinoma [64, 65].

Chemotherapy seems to enhance the negative effects of radiation for childhood solid tumors such as Wilms tumor [66–68]. For instance, Breslow and colleagues found a SIR of 36 for second cancer following therapy involving doxorubicin and more than 35 Gy of radiation for Wilms tumor [60]. This fact has essentially shaped the main preventive strategy, namely, to continue efforts to limit the use of intensive chemotherapy and radiation therapy, especially in combination. A French study summed up the challenge with respect to chemotherapy: 'to minimize the mutagenic effects of these drugs by diminishing cumulative doses without losing the therapeutic benefits' [69]. Apart from such adjustments, close surveillance must continue to be maintained in order to facilitate early diagnosis and treatment for any SPC [60, 70].

Notes and References

1 Dinu I, Liu Y, Leisenring W, et al: Prediction of second malignant neoplasm incidence in a large cohort of long-term survivors of childhood cancers. Pediatr Blood Cancer 2007, E-pub ahead of print.

2 Guibout C, Adjadj E, Rubino C, et al: Malignant breast tumors after radiotherapy for a first cancer during childhood. J Clin Oncol 2005;23:197–204.

3 Svahn-Tapper G, Garwicz S, Anderson H, et al: Radiation dose and relapse are predictors for development of second malignant solid tumors after cancer in childhood and adolescence: a population-based case-control study in the five Nordic countries. Acta Oncol 2006;45:438–448.

4 Jazbec J, Todorovski L, Jereb B: Classification tree analysis of second neoplasms in survivors of childhood cancer. BMC Cancer 2007;7:27.

5 Henderson TO, Whitton J, Stovall M, et al: Secondary sarcomas in childhood cancer survivors: a report from the Childhood Cancer Survivor Study. J Natl Cancer Inst 2007;99:300–308.

6 Guerin S, Hawkins M, Shamsaldin A, et al: Treatment-adjusted predisposition to second malignant neoplasms after a solid cancer in childhood: a case-control study. J Clin Oncol 2007;25:2833–2839.

7 Guerin S, Dupuy A, Anderson H, et al: Radiation dose as a risk factor for malignant melanoma following childhood cancer. Eur J Cancer 2003;39: 2379–2386.

8 Perkins JL, Liu Y, Mitby PA, et al: Nonmelanoma skin cancer in survivors of childhood and adolescent cancer: a report from the childhood cancer survivor study. J Clin Oncol 2005;23:3733–3741.

9 Neglia JP, Robison LL, Stovall M, et al: New primary neoplasms of the central nervous system in survivors of childhood cancer: a report from the Childhood Cancer Survivor Study. J Natl Cancer Inst 2006;98:1528–1537.

10 Jenkinson HC, Winter DL, Marsden HB, et al: A study of soft tissue sarcomas after childhood cancer in Britain. Br J Cancer 2007;97:695–699.

11 Inskip PD, Curtis RE: New malignancies following childhood cancer in the United States, 1973–2002. Int J Cancer 2007;121:2233–2240.

12 Lawless SC, Verma P, Green DM, et al: Mortality experiences among 15+ year survivors of childhood and adolescent cancers. Pediatr Blood Cancer 2007;48:333–338.

13 Skinner R, Wallace WH, Levitt G: Long-term follow-up of children treated for cancer: why is it necessary, by whom, where and how? Arch Dis Child 2007;92: 257–260.

14 Ng SK, Mackay S, Seymour JF: Surveillance of second cancer after previous childhood cancer treatment. Aust Fam Physician 2007;36:643–645.

15 Metayer C, Lynch CF, Clarke EA, et al: Second cancers among long-term survivors of Hodgkin's disease diagnosed in childhood and adolescence. J Clin Oncol 2000;18:2435–2443.
16 Lin HM, Teitell MA: Second malignancy after treatment of pediatric Hodgkin disease. J Pediatr Hematol Oncol 2005;27:28–36.
17 Bhatia S, Yasui Y, Robison LL, et al: High risk of subsequent neoplasms continues with extended follow-up of childhood Hodgkin's disease: report from the Late Effects Study Group. J Clin Oncol 2003;21: 4386–4394.
18 Maule M, Scelo G, Pastore G, et al: Risk of second malignant neoplasms after childhood leukemia and lymphoma: an international study. J Natl Cancer Inst 2007;99:790–800.
19 Schellong G, Riepenhausen M, Creutzig U, et al: Low risk of secondary leukemias after chemotherapy without mechlorethamine in childhood Hodgkin's disease. German-Austrian Pediatric Hodgkin's Disease Group. J Clin Oncol 1997;15:2247–2253.
20 Gray (symbol: Gy) is the measurement unit of the absorption of radiation energy: 1 Gy is the absorption of 1 J of radiation energy by 1 kg of matter.
21 Long-Term Follow-Up Guidelines for Survivors of Childhood, Adolescent, and Young Adult Cancers. Bethesda, CureSearch Children's Oncology Group, 2006.www.survivorshipguidelines.org/pdf/LTFU Guidelines. pdf (accessed December 2007).
22 Rubino C, Cailleux AF, De Vathaire F, et al: Thyroid cancer after radiation exposure. Eur J Cancer 2002;38: 645–647.
23 Schwartz CL: Special issues in pediatric Hodgkin's disease. Eur J Haematol 2005;66:55–62.
24 Friedmann AM, Hudson MM, Weinstein HJ, et al: Treatment of unfavorable childhood Hodgkin's disease with VEPA and low-dose, involved-field radiation. J Clin Oncol 2002;20:3088–3094.
25 Bhatia S: Late effects among survivors of leukemia during childhood and adolescence. Blood Cells Mol Dis 2003;31:84–92.
26 Colby-Graham MF, Chordas C: The childhood leukemias. J Pediatr Nurs 2003;18:87–95.
27 Suarez CR, Bertolone SJ, Raj AB, et al: Second malignant neoplasms in childhood acute lymphoblastic leukemia: primitive neuroectodermal tumor of the chest wall with germline p53 mutation as a second malignant neoplasm. Am J Hematol 2004;76:52–56.
28 Bhatia S, Sather HN, Pabustan OB, et al: Low incidence of second neoplasms among children diagnosed with acute lymphoblastic leukemia after 1983. Blood 2002;99:4257–4264.
29 Neglia JP, Friedman DL, Yasui Y, et al: Second malignant neoplasms in five-year survivors of childhood cancer: childhood cancer survivor study. J Natl Cancer Inst 2001;93:618–629.
30 Kowalczyk J, Nurzynska-Flak J, Armata J, et al: Incidence and clinical characteristics of second malignant neoplasms in children: a multicenter study of a polish pediatric leukemia/lymphoma group. Med Sci Monit 2004;10:CR117–CR122.
31 Acute nonlymphocytic leukemia.
32 Hijiya N, Hudson MM, Lensing S, et al: Cumulative incidence of secondary neoplasms as a first event after childhood acute lymphoblastic leukemia. JAMA 2007;297:1207–1215.
33 Maniar TN, Braunstein I, Keefe S, et al: Childhood ALL and second neoplasms. Cancer Biol Ther 2007; 6:1525–1531.
34 Goshen Y, Stark B, Kornreich L, et al: High incidence of meningioma in cranial irradiated survivors of childhood acute lymphoblastic leukemia. Pediatr Blood Cancer 2007;49:294–297.
35 Shusterman S, Meadows AT: Long term survivors of childhood leukemia. Curr Opin Hematol 2000;7: 217–222.
36 Oeffinger KC, Eshelman DA, Tomlinson GE, et al: Providing primary care for long-term survivors of childhood acute lymphoblastic leukemia. J Fam Pract 2000;49:1133–1146.
37 Walter AW, Hancock ML, Pui CH, et al: Secondary brain tumors in children treated for acute lymphoblastic leukemia at St Jude Children's Research Hospital. J Clin Oncol 1998;16:3761–3767.
38 Prasannan L, Pu A, Hoff P, et al: Parotid carcinoma as a second malignancy after treatment of childhood acute lymphoblastic leukemia. J Pediatr Hematol Oncol 1999;21:535–538.
39 Sasadeusz J, Kelly H, Szer J, et al: Abnormal cervical cytology in bone marrow transplant recipients. Bone Marrow Transplant 2001;28:393–397.
40 Libra M, Gloghini A, De Re V, et al: Aggressive forms of non-Hodgkin's lymphoma in two patients bearing coinfection of Epstein-Barr and hepatitis C viruses. Int J Oncol 2005;26:945–950.
41 Zeller GX, De Sutter E: A numerical overview of various forms of retinoblastoma. Klin Monatsbl Augenheilkd 1991;198:81–82.
42 A trilateral version involves an intracranial neuroblastic tumo, typically a pinealoblastoma.
43 Li FP: Familial cancer syndromes and clusters. Curr Probl Cancer 1990;14:73–114.
44 Kaye FJ, Harbour JW: For whom the bell tolls: susceptibility to common adult cancers in retinoblastoma survivors. J Natl Cancer Inst 2004;96:342–343.
45 Germline mutations are found in every cell descended from the zygote to which that mutant gamete contributed. If an adult is successfully produced, every one of its body (or somatic) cells will contain the mutation. The same is true of the gametes;so if the host is able to become a parent, that mutation will pass down to a new generation.

46 Fletcher O, Easton D, Anderson K, et al: Lifetime risks of common cancers among retinoblastoma survivors. J Natl Cancer Inst 2004;96:357–363.
47 Watts P: Retinoblastoma: clinical features and current concepts in management. J Ind Med Assoc 2003;101:464–466, 468.
48 Moll AC, Imhof SM, Bouter LM, et al: Second primary tumors in patients with retinoblastoma: a review of the literature. Ophthalmol Genet 1997;18: 27–34.
49 Mohney BG, Robertson DM, Schomberg PJ, et al: Second nonocular tumors in survivors of heritable retinoblastoma and prior radiation therapy. Am J Ophthalmol 1998;126:269–277.
50 Eng C, Li FP, Abramson DH, et al: Mortality from second tumors among long-term survivors of retinoblastoma. J Natl Cancer Inst 1993;85:1121–1128.
51 Kleinerman RA, Tucker MA, Abramson DH, et al: Risk of soft tissue sarcomas by individual subtype in survivors of hereditary retinoblastoma. J Natl Cancer Inst 2007;99:24–31.
52 Draper GJ, Sanders BM, Brownbill PA, et al: Patterns of risk of hereditary retinoblastoma and applications to genetic counselling. Br J Cancer 1992;66:211–219.
53 Kleinerman RA, Tucker MA, Tarone RE, et al: Risk of new cancers after radiotherapy in long-term survivors of retinoblastoma: an extended follow-up. J Clin Oncol 2005;23:2272–2279.
54 Wong FL, Boice JD Jr, Abramson DH, et al: Cancer incidence after retinoblastoma: radiation dose and sarcoma risk. JAMA 1997;278:1262–1267.
55 Paulino AC: Malignant neoplasms after treatment for metachronous bilateral Wilms' tumor: a literature review. Pediatr Hematol Oncol 1999;16: 533–538.
56 Weirich A, Ludwig R, Graf N, et al: Survival in nephroblastoma treated according to the trial and study SIOP-9/GPOH with respect to relapse and morbidity. Ann Oncol 2004;15:808–820.
57 Li FP, Yan JC, Sallan S, et al: Second neoplasms after Wilms' tumor in childhood. J Natl Cancer Inst 1983; 71:1205–1209.
58 Treated by radiotherapy.
59 Breslow NE, Norkool PA, Olshan A, et al: Second malignant neoplasms in survivors of Wilms' tumor: a report from the National Wilms' Tumor Study. J Natl Cancer Inst 1988;80:592–595.
60 Breslow NE, Takashima JR, Whitton JA, et al: Second malignant neoplasms following treatment for Wilm's tumor: a report from the National Wilms' Tumor Study Group. J Clin Oncol 1995;13: 1851–1859.
61 Carli M, Frascella E, Tournade MF, et al: Second malignant neoplasms in patients treated on SIOP Wilms tumour studies and trials 1, 2, 5, and 6. Med Pediatr Oncol 1997;29:239–244.
62 Cherullo EE, Ross JH, Kay R, et al: Renal neoplasms in adult survivors of childhood Wilms tumor. J Urol 2001;165:2013–2016; discussion 2016–2017.
63 Evans AE, Norkool P, Evans I, et al: Late effects of treatment for Wilms' tumor: a report from the National Wilms' Tumor Study Group. Cancer 1991; 67:331–336.
64 Beales IL, Scott HJ: Adenocarcinoma of the duodenum with a duodeno-colic fistula occurring after childhood Wilms' cancer. Postgrad Med J 1994;70: 933–936.
65 Densmore TL, Langer JC, Molleston JP, et al: Colorectal adenocarcinoma as a second malignant neoplasm following Wilms' tumor and rhabdomyosarcoma. Med Pediatr Oncol 1996;27:556–560.
66 Haddy N, Le Deley MC, Samand A, et al: Role of radiotherapy and chemotherapy in the risk of secondary leukaemia after a solid tumour in childhood. Eur J Cancer 2006;42:2757–2764.
67 Guerin S, Guibout C, Shamsaldin A, et al: Concomitant chemo-radiotherapy and local dose of radiation as risk factors for second malignant neoplasms after solid cancer in childhood: a case-control study. Int J Cancer 2006;120:96–102.
68 Menu-Branthomme A, Rubino C, Shamsaldin A, et al: Radiation dose, chemotherapy and risk of soft tissue sarcoma after solid tumours during childhood. Int J Cancer 2004;110:87–93.
69 Le Deley MC, Leblanc T, Shamsaldin A, et al: Risk of secondary leukemia after a solid tumor in childhood according to the dose of epipodophyllotoxins and anthracyclines: a case-control study by the Societe Francaise d'Oncologie Pediatrique. J Clin Oncol 2003;21:1074–1081.
70 Paulino AC, Wen BC, Brown CK, et al: Late effects in children treated with radiation therapy for Wilms' tumor. Int J Radiat Oncol Biol Phys 2000; 46:1239–1246.

Krueger H, McLean D, Williams D: The Prevention of Second Primary Cancers.
Prog Exp Tumor Res. Basel, Karger, 2008, vol 40, pp 135–137

15

Summary of Significant SPC Associations

As a final summary of our literature review, we offer 3 tables itemizing the SPCs with excess incidence based on the 'index' studies outlined in the monograph (fig. 3–5). The first 2 tables cover all cancer cases, while the third table focuses on pediatric cancers. On the first 2 tables, the first primary cancers are ranked based on the estimated incidence rate. On the first table, the SPCs are also sorted based on estimated number of individuals with the cancer. On the second and third tables, the SPCs are ranked based on 5-year patient survival rates associated with each cancer.

To our knowledge, the following tables represent the first comprehensive synthesis of data that looks at all of the most relevant first primaries and associated second primaries. Two other recent papers did accomplish something similar, but the analysis was limited to a single cancer registry and thus generally was based on smaller pools of each first primary than we have accessed. As a consequence, the range of identified significant associations was much more limited. These 2 reports also deviated from our analysis in other important ways, as we note below.

In an examination of the South Australian Cancer Registry, Heard et al. [1] detected 20 SPC categories in significant excess following a first primary, including 3 types associated with lip cancer (a site we did not specifically focus upon due to limited data in the wider literature). Unfortunately, their study did not report the actual SIRs when 'same month' diagnoses were excluded, data that would have allowed a better comparison with the true SPC information we have assembled.

Bajdik et al. [2] considered cancer cases in the province of British Columbia, Canada, between 1970 and 2004. Rather than SPCs per se, the authors focused on multiple primaries, that is, associations between 2 or more cancers in 1 patient, regardless of temporal directionality. Among female patients, they found 1 association between 2 cancers with a SIR higher than 2; there were 8 such relevant cancer pairs among men.

Notes and References

1 Heard A, Roder D, Luke C: Multiple primary cancers of separate organ sites: implications for research and cancer control. Cancer Causes Control 2005;16:475–481.

2 Bajdik CD, Abanto ZU, Spinelli JJ, et al: Identifying related cancer types based on their incidence among people with multiple cancers. Emerg Themes Epidemiol 2006;3:17.

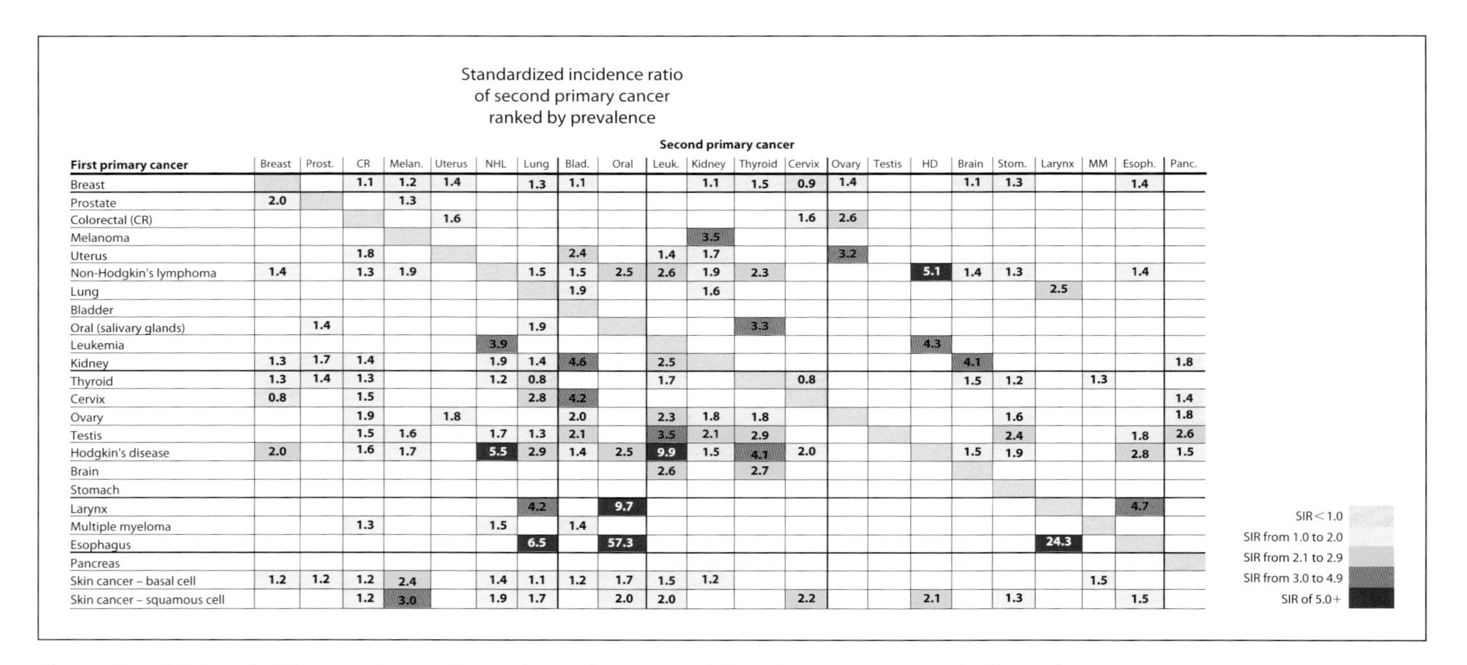

Standardized incidence ratio of second primary cancer ranked by prevalence

First primary cancer	Second primary cancer: Breast	Prost.	CR	Melan.	Uterus	NHL	Lung	Blad.	Oral	Leuk.	Kidney	Thyroid	Cervix	Ovary	Testis	HD	Brain	Stom.	Larynx	MM	Esoph.	Panc.
Breast			1.1	1.2	1.4		1.3	1.1			1.1	1.5	0.9	1.4			1.1	1.3			1.4	
Prostate	2.0			1.3																		
Colorectal (CR)					1.6								1.6	2.6								
Melanoma											3.5											
Uterus			1.8					2.4		1.4	1.7			3.2								
Non-Hodgkin's lymphoma	1.4		1.3	1.9			1.5	1.5	2.5	2.6	1.9	2.3				5.1	1.4	1.3			1.4	
Lung								1.9			1.6								2.5			
Bladder																						
Oral (salivary glands)		1.4					1.9					3.3										
Leukemia						3.9										4.3						
Kidney	1.3	1.7	1.4			1.9	1.4	4.6		2.5							4.1					1.8
Thyroid	1.3	1.4	1.3			1.2	0.8			1.7			0.8				1.5	1.2		1.3		
Cervix	0.8		1.5				2.8	4.2														1.4
Ovary			1.9		1.8			2.0		2.3	1.8	1.8						1.6				1.8
Testis			1.5	1.6		1.7	1.3	2.1		3.5	2.1	2.9						2.4			1.8	2.6
Hodgkin's disease	2.0		1.6	1.7		5.5	2.9	1.4	2.5	9.9	1.5	4.1	2.0				1.5	1.9			2.8	1.5
Brain										2.6		2.7										
Stomach																						
Larynx							4.2		9.7												4.7	
Multiple myeloma			1.3			1.5		1.4														
Esophagus							6.5		57.3										24.3			
Pancreas																						
Skin cancer – basal cell	1.2	1.2	1.2	2.4		1.4	1.1	1.2	1.7	1.5	1.2									1.5		
Skin cancer – squamous cell			1.2	3.0		1.9	1.7		2.0	2.0			2.2			2.1		1.3			1.5	

Fig. 3. SIR of SPC ranked by prevalence. CR = Colorectal; HD = Hodgkin's disease; MM = multiple myeloma.

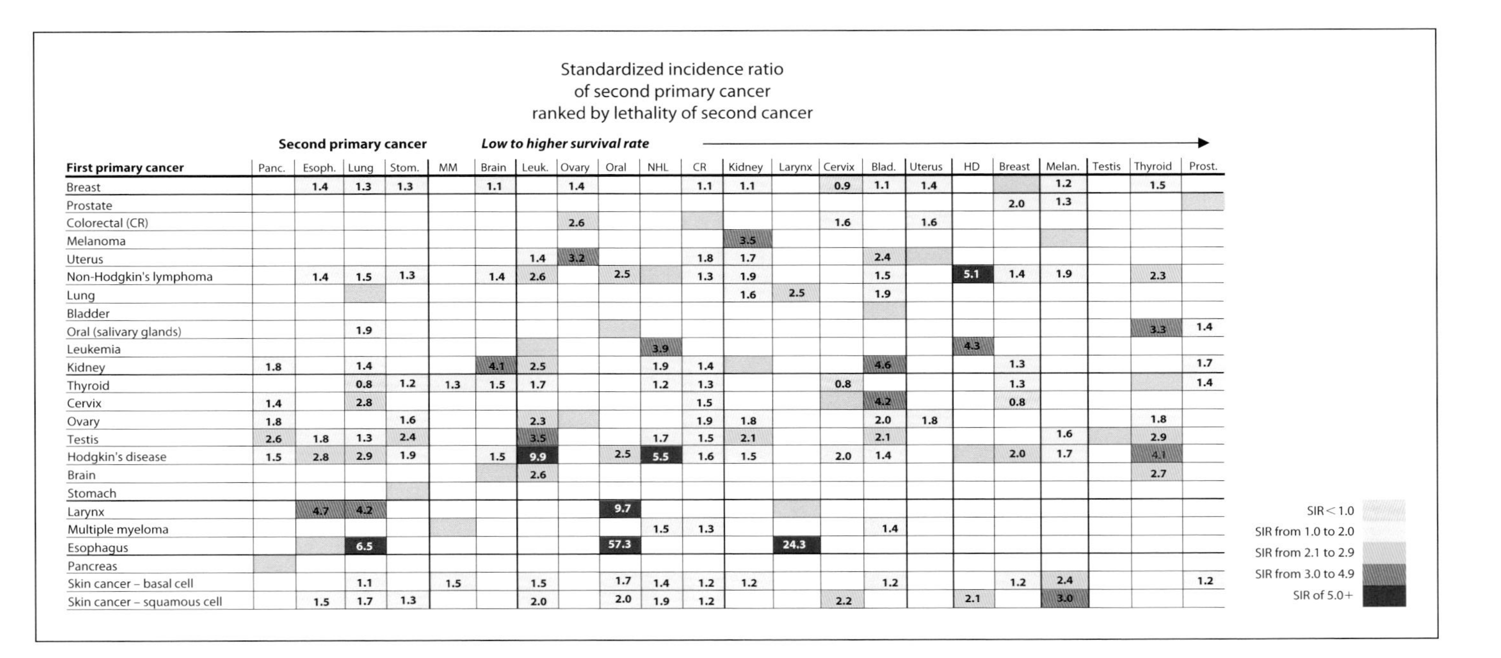

Standardized incidence ratio of second primary cancer ranked by lethality of second cancer

Second primary cancer — *Low to higher survival rate* →

First primary cancer	Panc.	Esoph.	Lung	Stom.	MM	Brain	Leuk.	Ovary	Oral	NHL	CR	Kidney	Larynx	Cervix	Blad.	Uterus	HD	Breast	Melan.	Testis	Thyroid	Prost.
Breast		1.4	1.3	1.3		1.1		1.4			1.1	1.1		0.9	1.1	1.4			1.2		1.5	
Prostate																		2.0	1.3			
Colorectal (CR)								2.6						1.6		1.6						
Melanoma												3.5										
Uterus							1.4	3.2			1.8	1.7			2.4							
Non-Hodgkin's lymphoma		1.4	1.5	1.3		1.4	2.6		2.5		1.3	1.9			1.5		5.1	1.4	1.9		2.3	
Lung												1.6	2.5		1.9							
Bladder																						
Oral (salivary glands)			1.9																		3.3	1.4
Leukemia										3.9							4.3					
Kidney	1.8		1.4			4.1	2.5			1.9	1.4				4.6			1.3				1.7
Thyroid			0.8	1.2	1.3	1.5	1.7			1.2	1.3			0.8				1.3				1.4
Cervix	1.4		2.8								1.5				4.2			0.8				
Ovary	1.8			1.6			2.3				1.9	1.8			2.0	1.8					1.8	
Testis	2.6	1.8	1.3	2.4			3.5			1.7	1.5	2.1			2.1				1.6		2.9	
Hodgkin's disease	1.5	2.8	2.9	1.9		1.5	9.9		2.5	5.5	1.6	1.5		2.0	1.4			2.0	1.7		4.1	
Brain							2.6														2.7	
Stomach																						
Larynx		4.7	4.2						9.7													
Multiple myeloma										1.5	1.3				1.4							
Esophagus			6.5						57.3				24.3									
Pancreas																						
Skin cancer – basal cell			1.1		1.5		1.5		1.7	1.4	1.2	1.2			1.2			1.2	2.4			1.2
Skin cancer – squamous cell		1.5	1.7	1.3			2.0		2.0	1.9	1.2			2.2			2.1		3.0			

Fig. 4. SIR of SPC ranked by lethality of second cancer. MM = Multiple myeloma; CR = colorectal; HD = Hodgkin's disease.

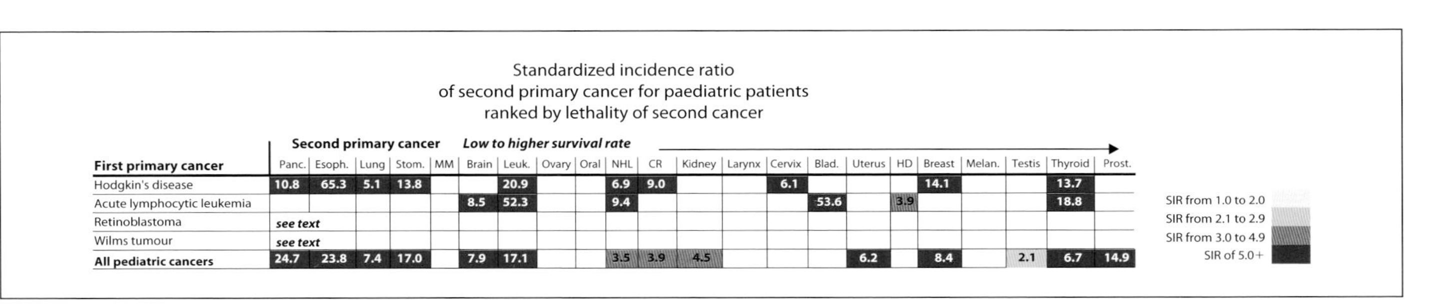

Standardized incidence ratio of second primary cancer for paediatric patients ranked by lethality of second cancer

Second primary cancer — *Low to higher survival rate* →

First primary cancer	Panc.	Esoph.	Lung	Stom.	MM	Brain	Leuk.	Ovary	Oral	NHL	CR	Kidney	Larynx	Cervix	Blad.	Uterus	HD	Breast	Melan.	Testis	Thyroid	Prost.
Hodgkin's disease	10.8	65.3	5.1	13.8			20.9			6.9	9.0			6.1				14.1			13.7	
Acute lymphocytic leukemia						8.5	52.3			9.4					53.6		3.9				18.8	
Retinoblastoma	*see text*																					
Wilms tumour	*see text*																					
All pediatric cancers	24.7	23.8	7.4	17.0		7.9	17.1			3.5	3.9	4.5				6.2		8.4		2.1	6.7	14.9

Fig. 5. SIR of SPC for pediatric patients ranked by lethality of second cancer. MM = Multiple myeloma; CR = colorectal; HD = Hodgkin's disease.

Krueger H, McLean D, Williams D: The Prevention of Second Primary Cancers.
Prog Exp Tumor Res. Basel, Karger, 2008, vol 40, pp 138–144

16

Population Health Priorities

From a population health and prevention perspective, the critical initial question is whether SPC is of much concern at all. Based on large patient registries, the excess risk for SPCs taken together can be characterized as relatively low. When not focusing on the pediatric population, the statistically significant results for the SIR for second cancers combined ranges from 1.06 to about 1.50. In some population-based studies, the risk of SPC was not elevated at all. It would be easy to follow the conclusion of Finnish epidemiologists in 1995: 'subsequent neoplasms among cancer patients do not pose a major public-health problem' [1]. They maintained, as we have noted in our monograph, that there already is legitimate and well-established focus on SPC at the level of therapy and clinical follow-up of individual patients. With this perspective applied at the broadest level, population level prevention of SPC would be of only modest interest.

We hope that our monograph has made it clear that overly conservative conclusions about prevention of second cancers may be hasty. It is true that, measured against the spectrum of all cancers, and especially against malignancies of high incidence, the aggregate phenomenon of SPC may not seem to be alarming. But when we narrow the focus to specific cancers or specific age groups, the story becomes very different.

A Program for Pediatric Cancer Survivors

We have observed that the risks of SPC are substantially elevated following a history of pediatric cancer. For instance, multiple studies based on large samples revealed that there can be up to an 8-fold increased risk of SPC following Wilms tumor; the excess risk following pediatric Hodgkin's disease is of a similar magnitude, and even taking all childhood cancers together appears to yield an overall SIR between 5 and 6. Another example was provided by a very recent study that added to our understanding of skin cancer following pediatric cancer; it revealed that the SIR for the basal cell carcinomas of the skin approaches 12 in pediatric cancer survivors (mostly attributable to the effects of ionizing radiation used in therapy) [2].

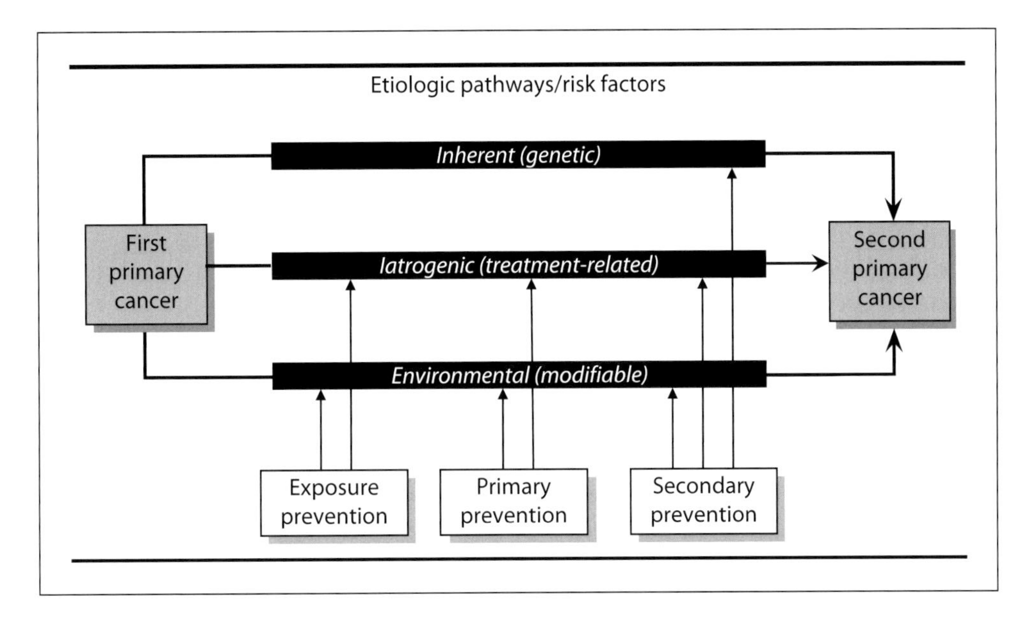

Fig. 6. Etiologic pathways/risk factors.

There is clear support for a population level screening and prevention program for pediatric cancer survivors. From a prevention point of view, our monograph has underlined several implications for the follow-up care of survivors of childhood cancer. The following list offers the foundation for an appropriate protocol in this high-risk cohort.

Risk assessment: Identify the SPCs with significant excess risk following a first primary; the aim is to focus and intensify prevention efforts as warranted.

Exposure prevention (1): As noted in figure 6, when a SPC of concern is iatrogenic (that is, therapy induced), an exposure prevention strategy would be to develop and deploy alternate, safer therapies or protocols for the treatment of the pediatric cancer. Of course, given the time required for such research, this sort of prevention commitment must happen long before the presentation of the first primary.

Exposure prevention (2): When the SPC of concern has a modifiable (usually behavioral) risk factor, we should encourage people not to take up the behavior in the first place. For example, there is a real opportunity in motivating young cancer patients towards not initiating tobacco use or avoiding sexual practices that expose them to viruses that cause cancer [3]. Such prevention efforts must occur at both personal and societal levels.

Primary prevention (1): As seen in fig. 3, the first form of primary prevention involves intervening to reverse modifiable risk factors of the SPC (for example, smoking cessation or maintaining a healthy diet). Again, this can happen at a personal/behavioral level or by removing carcinogens from the general environment (for example, preventing exposure to second-hand smoke through regulations). Another recently launched mode of primary prevention that will have a significant effect on certain types of SPC (for example, cervical and oral) is population-wide HPV vaccination, where the impact of a common etiologic agent (in this case, a virus) is interrupted.

Primary prevention (2): Chemoprevention (if an effective approach is available) should be applied to avoid, arrest or reverse the development of a SPC. This includes the use of radiation chemoprotectants. Again, actually developing/testing new agents is a prevention measure that must predate the presentation of the second primary. Such a program for pediatric cancer survivors can be based in an adult medical center (as the cancers tend to occur in adults) or in the community. Ideally, primary care physicians will be reminded through various practice tools of particular risks and appropriate interventions. Information systems can be tailored to each patient's cancer and the specific therapeutic agents to which they have been exposed. Computerization permits cost-effective notification for both the patient and the physician, on a regular basis.

Secondary prevention: Surveillance and early detection of SPC. As the latency period for cancer development can be very long, this sort of follow-up sometimes must be maintained for decades. Programs involving at least an annual clinical assessment, including a skin exam and cervical cytology, may be appropriate.

Genetic assessment: If a genetic linkage between the first and second primaries is known, or if other genetic susceptibility or molecular precursors of disease are detected, then any of the above measures that are appropriate must be pursued in an intensified and/or targeted way. For example, as an expression of so-called personalized medicine, chemoprevention may one day be directed at specific molecular defects. This is the most advanced scenario on the horizon, at least until the day when effective interventions directly influencing the genome are developed.

A Program for Survivors of Adult-Onset Cancer

Risk assessment is the starting point with respect to adult-onset first primaries. The key question is: what is the excess burden of cancers that may be expected following a first primary cancer? This monograph has focused on assembling data to assist with answering this very question for adult and pediatric patients. An important difference with adult cancers is that there are simply so many more of them on the watch list. We saw that the pediatric cancers associated with the greatest excess risk or otherwise of interest could be numbered on 1 hand: Hodgkin's disease, acute lymphocytic leukemia, retinoblastoma and Wilms tumor. In contrast, we have seen that there are a large number of adult-onset first primary cancers that are associated with a significant excess risk of SPC and in some cases generate a substantial absolute burden of 'unexpected' cancer cases.

A convenient inventory of SPC associations was already provided in the summary in the preceding chapter of this monograph. There are many ways to order such information. One possibility is to organize the first primary according to prevalence (which we have done). Another possibility is to arrange the SPC according to decreasing mortality rate or increasing survival (which we provided in the second summary table). A prevalence perspective is important at the population level; while approaches related to mortality/survival may mean more to the individual patient and their caregivers.

While the main interest of health system managers is population health, the phenomenon of SPC should never underestimate the felt reality of the individual human being. A 2006 study by Deimling et al. [4] added to the growing literature on the psychosocial aspect of cancer survivorship. Even if the devastation of a second cancer is forestalled, there are significant levels of anxiety and even depression related to the threat of new cancers and the concomitant reduction in life expectancy.

To increase the health of a population and improve the quality of life of individual cancer survivors, it is important to assess the current state of prevention measures, and to encourage more progress where needed. The overall 'protocol' for adult-onset cancers is similar to that laid out for pediatric patients above, that is, a combination of exposure as well as primary and secondary prevention efforts that takes into account any relevant risk factors.

We should note that sometimes a threatened SPC shares 1 or more inherent or environmental risk factors with the original cancer. This really calls for very little adjustment to existing prevention mandates. This is clear in the event of inherent factors such as genetic makeup over which there is little or no control in the first place. But even in the case of behavioral risk factors, the plan may remain fairly static. For example, a recommendation to stop smoking applies equally before and after a tobacco-related first primary when the SPC prevention focus entails another tobacco-related tumor.

In this light, 2 practical implications of shared risk factors may be further elucidated:

(1) In the case of modifiable (especially behavioral) factors, the cancer survivor may already be educated about or engaged in primary prevention measures (or employers may be making the workplace safer, etc.). In this way, the prevention efforts with respect to the SPC become intertwined with a generalized prevention message and strategy, and thus may feel less like a special initiative (which may or may not make the job harder for health professionals). The best scenario would be for the 'threat' of a SPC to motivate an intensification of standard prevention measures.

(2) In the case of a hereditary or familial pattern or a long-term exposure to a carcinogen common to first and second cancers, certain cells, especially in mucosal epithelia, may be preconditioned for carcinoma development (some theorists ominously refer to this as 'condemned mucosa syndrome') [5]. This means that any new cancer may need to be distinguished from the 'partially clonal' dysplasia and malignant neoplasms that some researchers do not consider to be true SPC at all. Once again, the basic clinical or preventive measures are ultimately not affected by the precise type of multiple cancer emerging in such settings. Smoking cessation, healthy weight, calorie-burning exercise, proper diet, limiting

sun exposure and, in the case of oral/esophageal cancer, reduction in excessive drinking are almost always the first and most vital public health and patient commitments.

The preceding point, especially the list of prevention maneuvers, makes plain something that has been implicit all along: the key efforts relayed to behavioral risk factors that should be brought to bear to reduce SPC development coincide precisely with the 'five primary preventable risk factors' [6] recommended as the path to preventing up to 50% of all types of malignancies, no matter the order in which they occur in a patient.

Prevention Primer: SRS for SPC

The ultimate 'million dollar' question is whether targeted and perhaps unique strategies can be brought to bear to reduce the excess burden connected to SPC. To be of extra benefit, the effort has to extend beyond smoking cessation, because clearly that intervention is being driven home (or should be) for *all citizens at all times* anyway.

The volume of information presented in this monograph seems to support a disconcertingly limited amount of precise guidance for either clinicians or population health specialists. The basic prevention program for SPC can be summarized under the following 3 headings (each contributing to our proposed acronym, SRS).

Safest Treatment Possible: The first strategy involves opting for safer therapeutic agents or regimens, where safety is guided not just by short-term toxicity but by late effects as well. This is especially important in treating pediatric cancers, where therapies are now so successful that long survival is the norm. We reiterate here that a great deal of the SPC story is a by-product of the dramatic improvement in pediatric cancer therapies, cure rates and patient survival in recent decades. To some extent, this fundamental, somewhat ironic conclusion also applies to adult-onset malignancies: more cancer patients are simply surviving long enough these days to actually develop a second primary. The onus on medical professionals is to seek to reduce this risk as much as possible, beginning with using the most favorable therapy, that is the one that yields the best balance of risks and benefits.

Risk Factor Reduction: The next step involves encouraging patients to modify relevant SPC risk factors that have a behavioral component. This can involve one-to-one clinical efforts or wider health promotion programs. We would include under this category all public policies that make healthy choices the easy choice, as well as eliminating passive carcinogen exposures (for example, second-hand smoke, occupational chemicals and pollution). As we have already stated, the good and bad news is that there is nothing particularly unique about these efforts; this means that SPC prevention categories overlap greatly with general health initiatives such as smoking cessation. Having said that, the excess risk attached to a tobacco-related SPC, for instance, could lead to targeted and intensified efforts to eliminate tobacco use among a particular subset of patients. Support for individualized counseling and nicotine replacement therapy may be strongly cost-effective in this subset of cancer survivors. It is important to realize that simply addressing any behavioral risk factors generally holds out greater hope than more complex scenarios, including current chemoprevention options for SPC [7].

Surveillance and Early Intervention: A final component of the prevention armamentarium is surveillance for SPC, to facilitate early detection and treatment [8]. Again, this category is not necessarily unique to SPC. It is often overshadowed by general population programs, such as screening mammography and cervical screening. However, information about second cancers and specific SIR data may certainly guide surveillance protocols tailored to the SPC in question and inform decisions about specialized treatment. Such follow-up should always be aimed at earlier diagnosis of and response to SPCs in high-risk patients.

A Vital Research Horizon

The rather limited scope represented by the preceding strategies points to what may be the most important priority in a state-of-the-art prevention program, namely, ongoing research into SPC [9]. This includes development and testing of new therapies for the first primary cancer, greater understanding of modifiable risk factors that account for excess risk of a SPC and improvements in surveillance techniques [10]. Stratification of results derived from increasingly sophisticated cancer registries (taking into account, for example, age and stage of first primary diagnosis, follow-up period, gender, first primary therapy method and other risk factors) will permit more finely tuned approaches to primary and secondary prevention. It might also shed light on the rare instances of a seemingly protective effect for SPC following certain first primaries.

The most cutting edge investigations will probably focus on the genetic underpinnings of second cancer occurrence. Whether familial or sporadic, being able to detect the presence of a genetic defect will allow the most precise treatment and follow-up protocols and hold out hope for substantial reduction of SPC population risks and improved quality of life for individualized cancer survivors [11]. We suggest that in the next decade there will be many examples of this sort of personalized cancer control program.

1 Sankila R, Pukkala E, Teppo L: Risk of subsequent malignant neoplasms among 470,000 cancer patients in Finland, 1953–1991. Int J Cancer 1995;60:464–470.

2 Levi F, Moeckli R, Randumbison L, et al: Skin cancer in survivors of childhood and adolescent cancer. Eur J Cancer 2006;42:656–659.

3 The area of sexual health helps to illustrate that primary prevention is a more complex topic than people sometimes realize. Primary prevention actually comes in 3 levels: absolute prevention of exposure, reducing the risk of exposure or reducing the risk of a negative effect due to exposure. These 3 approaches may be illustrated in terms of sexual health in the following hierarchy of measures: abstinence, condom usage and vaccination.

4 Deimling GT, Bowman KF, Sterns S, et al: Cancer-related health worries and psychological distress among older adult, long-term cancer survivors. Psychooncology 2006;15:306–320.
5 Pillai MR, Nair MK: Development of a condemned mucosa syndrome and pathogenesis of human papillomavirus-associated upper aerodigestive tract and uterine cervical tumors. Exp Mol Pathol 2000; 69:233–241.
6 A convenient and effective summary of the 5 risk factors and the attendant prevention measures may be found in Cancer Prevention Facts. Vancouver , BC Cancer Agency, 2006. http://www.bccancer.bc.ca/NR/rdonlyres/483D2456-286B-46DA-A12D-69C8E081CCC5/18847/5GivesYouFiftyFeb06.pdf (accessed December 2007).
7 Mayne ST, Cartmel B: Chemoprevention of second cancers. Cancer Epidemiol Biomarkers Prev 2006;15: 2033–2037.
8 Vogel VG: Identifying and screening patients at risk of second cancers. Cancer Epidemiol Biomarkers Prev 2006;15:2027–2032.
9 Alberts DS: Second cancers are killing us! Cancer Epidemiol Biomarkers Prev 2006;15:2019.
10 Travis LB: The epidemiology of second primary cancers. Cancer Epidemiol Biomarkers Prev 2006; 15:2020–2026.
11 Travis LB, Rabkin CS, Brown LM, et al: Cancer survivorship – genetic susceptibility and second primary cancers: research strategies and recommendations. J Natl Cancer Inst 2006;98:15–25.

Dr. David I. McLean
Head, Cancer Prevention Programs, BC Cancer Agency
750 West Broadway Avenue
Vancouver, BC, V5Z 1H5 (Canada)
Tel. +1 604 877 6299, Fax +1 604 877 6212, E-Mail david.mclean@ubc.ca

Subject Index